The *ABSITE* Final Review

General Surgery In-Training Exam

Created by
MAURICIO SZUCHMACHER MD
MARIANA G.B.SZUCHMACHER MD
PRASHANT SUKHARAMWALA MD

Junior & Senior Edition

ISBN:1497300959
ISBN-13: 9781497300958

EDITORS-IN-CHIEF

Mauricio Szuchmacher, MD

Department of Vascular Surgery
North Shore-Long Island Jewish Health System
Hofstra School of Medicine
Manhasset, New York

Prashant Sukharamwala, MD

Department of Hepatopancreatobiliary Surgery
Florida Hospital
Tampa, Florida

GUEST EDITOR

K. V. Krishnasastry, MD FACS

Chief, Vascular and Endovascular Surgery
Fellowship Program Director
Vice-Chairman, Department of Surgery
Professor of Surgery at
Hofstra School of Medicine
North Shore-Long Island Jewish Health System

INTERNATIONAL EDITOR
Rossano K.A. Fiorelli, MD

Professor of Surgery
Chairman, Department of Surgery
Director, Post Graduate Medicine Program
Federal University Of State Of Rio de Janeiro

CONTRIBUTORS

Department of Vascular Surgery
North Shore-Long Island Jewish Health System
Hofstra School of Medicine

Rajeev Gupta, MD   **Omar Hamdallah**   **Shahin Pourrabani**
Vascular Surgery   Vascular Surgery   Vascular Surgery

Manhasset, New York

Northeast Ohio Medical University
Western Reserve Health Education
Northside Medical Center, Ohio

Abel Bello MD   **Tyler Bedford MD**   **Jonathan Thoes MD**
General Surgery   General Surgery   General Surgery

V. Yalamanchilli MD   **Sean Johnson MD**   **Michael Boyd MD**
General Surgery   General Surgery   General Surgery

Stephen Jones MD   **Ana Paula de O.**   **Gregg Tanner MD**
General Surgery   **Pereira MD**   General Surgery
                           General Surgery

Samuel Han MD   **Yashas Nathani MS**
General Surgery   **Melanie Nukala MD**   American University
                           General Surgery   of Antigua

DEDICATION

We dedicate this book to our families and to all of the amazing people who assisted with this project.
Without all of you we would not be successful in this journey!

DISCLAIMER

The purpose of this book is to assist surgical residents in the annual American Board of Surgery In training Exam.

The majority of the information can be found in major surgical textbooks, journal articles and websites. Main sources and suggested readings include, but are not limited to:

Current Surgical Therapy: 10ed (Current Therapy)
by John L. Cameron MD FACS FRCS FRCSI and Andrew M Cameron MD PhD (Jan 4, 2011)

Schwartz's Principles of Surgery, 9th Ed.
by F. Brunicardi, Dana Andersen, Timothy Billiar and David Dunn (Sep 11, 2009)

UpToDate®: www.uptodate.com

SCORE® www.surgicalcore.org

The authors do not have anything to disclose and have not been endorsed by the American Board of Surgery or American College of Surgeons.
No reproduction, copying, memorization, recall or reconstruction of the actual ABSITE examination was performed by any means to generate this question book. The authors have never had access to the ABSITE exams used by the American Board of Surgery Inc. other than to take the exam.

CONTENTS

ACKNOWLEDGMENTS

We acknowledge all of our families, mentors, students, residents, fellows, surgeons and specially, our patients.

Thank you also to those many others who contributed, directly and indirectly, to this work.

1. CELL BIOLOGY, HISTOLOGY AND WOUND HEALING

1) The most important cell to wound healing is:

    a) Platelet
    b) Macrophage
    c) Myofibroblasts
    d) Polymorphonucleocytes

    Overall, Macrophages are by far the most important cells
    because they secrete the **majority of the cytokines and
    growth factors** needed for wound healing. Platelets are the
    initial cell, followed by PMNs, macrophages,
    myofibroblasts and lymphocytes. **Answer B**.

2) The most prominent cell during the inflammatory phase is:

    a) Platelet
    b) Macrophage
    c) Myofibroblasts
    d) Polymorphonucleocytes

    The most predominant cells during the inflammatory
    phase are the macrophages, with highest levels around day
    2-3 after the initial insult. **Answer B**.

3) Platelets secret alpha granules important in beginning the
    wound healing process, including:

    a) Vascular Endothelial growth factor
    b) Transforming growth factor beta
    c) Tumor necrosis factor alpha
    d) Insulin growth factor

    TGF beta, PDGF, Platelet-activating factor, fibronectin,
    and serotonin are alpha granules secreted by platelets. **TGF
    beta** is an **angiogenesis** mediator. **Answer B**.

1

4) What day does collagen production begin:

   a) Day 3
   b) Day 7
   c) Day 21
   d) Immediately after initial insult

   Day 7 is when initial collagen, Type 3, is produced. This will later be broken down and replaced by Type 1, which is the major component of the extracellular matrix in skin. **Answer B.**

5) Which cell is primarily responsible for causing neovascularization:

   a) Fibroblasts
   b) Neutrophils
   c) Lymphocytes
   d) Macrophages

   Macrophages most important function is cell recruitment and activation via growth factors and cytokines. They secrete TGF beta, EGF, VEGF, and Insulin-like growth factor, regulating angiogenesis and matrix synthesis. They achieve significant number between days 2-4 and remain until wound healing is complete. **Answer D.**

6) Wound healing is not impaired in the following connective tissue disease:

   a) Marfan's syndrome
   b) Osteogenesis imperfecta
   c) Ehlers-Danlos Syndrome
   d) Acrodermatitis enteropathica

Marfan's syndrome does not delay wound healing because it affects the extracellular protein **fibrillin**, associated with elastic fibers. OI is associated with deficient Type I collagen and presents with osteopenia and joint laxity. ED is associated with deficiency on Type III collagen and AE is characterized by poor zinc absortion, impairing granulation tissue formation. **Answer A.**

7) Which of the following phases is not part of the normal healing process:

a) Inflammatory
b) Proliferative
c) Hypertrophic
d) Remodeling

The 3 main stages of wound healing are Inflammatory (0-2 weeks), Proliferative (3-6 weeks) and Remodeling (up to 1 year). **Answer C.**

8) Which of the following occurs in the proliferative phase:

a) Platelet degranulation
b) Initiation of collagen formation
c) Vasodilation
d) Increase tensile strength

During the proliferative phase, epithelialization, fibroblast proliferation and collagen production occurs. **Answer B.**

9) Which of the following occurs during the inflammatory phase:

a) Platelet degranulation
b) Vasoconstriction after 24hs
c) Vasodilation before 24hs
d) Decrease in capillary density

Important components of the inflammatory phase are **cellular recruitment and vascular permeability**. Platelet plug, vasoconstriction (first 24h) and vasodilation (24-48hs) also occur during this phase. **Answer A.**

10) Which of the following occurs during the remodeling phase:

   a) Fibroblasts proliferation
   b) Collagen cross-linking
   c) Decrease tensile strength
   d) Collagen equilibrium

   Remodeling is characterized by collagen maturation and wound contraction. Increase in **tensile strength and decreased fibroblasts** also occur in the remodeling phase. Approximately 80% of the original strength is achieved after 6 weeks. **Answer D.**

11) What is the correct order of cells arrive during the process of wound healing:

   a) PMNs, Macrophages, Platelets, Fibroblasts
   b) Macrophages, Platelets, Fibroblasts, PMNs
   c) Platelets, PMNs, Macrophages, Fibroblasts
   d) Fibroblasts, Macrophages, PMNs, Platelets

   Immediately after injury to the skin, **vasoconstriction** occurs to provide initial hemostasis. **Platelets aggregate** and degranulate, releasing essential growth factors and cytokines for **PMNs mobilization**. During the **inflammation phase**, maturation of blood-derived monocytes into **macrophages** occurs and this is followed by the epithelization/**fibroplasia phase**, consisted of **fibroblast proliferation**, and collagen production. **Answer C.**

12) Which of the following collagen predominates in keloid scars:

a) Type I
b) Type II
c) Type III
d) Type IV

Keloids and hypertrophic scars (HTS) are predominantly Type I collagen. **Keloids grow beyond** the margins of the original injury or scar. **HTS**s rise above the skin level but stay **within the confines** of the original wound and **often regress** over time. Keloids **excision** alone has a high recurrence rate, but decreases if **combined with** other modalities such as **intralesional steroid** injection, topical silicone sheets, radiation therapy, or pressure. **Answer A**.

13) Which of the following options describes the steroid effect on wound healing:

a) Increases cell migration to the wound
b) Is responsible for increasing selectins on cell surface
c) Causes vasoconstriction
d) Inhibits inflammatory cells and collagen synthesis

Steroids impair wound healing by interfering with **inflammation**, fibroblast proliferation, collagen **synthesis**, angiogenesis, wound contraction, and re-epithelialization. These effects are mediated by the antagonism of growth factors and cytokines. **Vitamin A restores** the inflammatory response and collagen synthesis. **Answer D**.

14) Which of the following is the most potent stimulator of the acute phase reactants:

a) IL-1
b) IL-2
c) IL-6
d) IL-10

IL-6 is the most potent stimulator of the acute phase reactants: C-reactive protein, Amyloid A, fibrinogen, haptoglobin, ceruloplasmin and C3. It is an inhibitor of Albumin and transferrin. Plasma levels of **IL-6 are proportional to the degree of injury** during, and it has **anti-inflammatory effects** through the inhibition of TNF and IL-1. **IL-10 inhibits** the secretion of **proinflammatory cytokines**, including TNF and IL-1. **Answer C.**

15) A septic patient is being monitored closely in the SICU. He continues to spike fevers, have elevated WBC count and tachycardia. Which of the following is most likely the mediator for his fever:

   a) IL-1
   b) IL-2
   c) IL-6
   d) IL-10

   IL-1 is synthesized by monocytes, macrophages, endothelial cells, and fibroblasts. Released **in response to inflammatory stimuli**, it mediates febrile response by **stimulating prostaglandin** activity **in the hypothalamus.** **IL-2** promotes T-lymphocyte proliferation, and IG production, explaining the **immunosuppressive effects** of IL-2 receptor blockade and pharmacological use for **organ transplantation. Answer A.**

16) Which of the following is the most potent stimulus for angiogenesis:

   a) VEGF
   b) Hypoxia
   c) EGF
   d) TGF-Beta

VEGF expression is regulated by hypoxia, providing a feedback mechanism to **reduced tissue oxygenation** via the **promotion of new blood vessel formation**. This is mediated by **hypoxia-inducible transcription factors** (HIF), which increase transcription of the VEGF gene. Cytokines such as EGF and TGF-beta also increase VEGF expression by different mechanisms. **Answer B.**

17) Which of the following is the most variable stage in the cell cycle:

    a) G1
    b) G2
    c) S
    d) M

The cell cycle is classically categorized into 4 distinct phases. Cells are generally most **radiosensitive** during **G_2 and in M** phase. **Answer A.**

Cell Cycle Phases	Features
G1	Synthesis of various enzymes, mainly for DNA replication. Duration is highly variable
S	Amount of DNA in the cell doubled. Duration is relatively constant among cells.
G2	Protein synthesis, lasts until the cell enters mitosis. Inhibition prevents the cell from undergoing mitosis.
M	Mitosis and cytokinesis. Cells that have stopped dividing enter the G_0 or quiescent phase.

18) Which of the following occurs after thyroxine is deiodinated to triiodothyronine:

a) Binds to a cytoplasm receptor, enter the nucleus and inhibits translation
b) Binds to cell membrane receptor, enter the cytoplasm and promotes translation
c) Enter the nucleus via active transport and promotes transcription
d) Inhibits messenger RNA after binding to a receptor in the nucleus

Thyroid hormones as well as steroids are **transcription factors. Thyroid hormone has it's receptor in the nucleus whereas steroid hormone receptor is in the cytoplasm.** T_4 is deiodinated to T_3 and enters the nucleus via active transport, where it binds to the thyroid hormone and leads to the transcription and translation of specific hormone genes. **Answer C.**

19) What is the mechanism of action of Nitric Oxide :

a) Inhibiting phosphodiesterase
b) Causing vasoconstriction
c) Increasing cAMP
d) Increasing cGMP

NO is a potent endogenous vasodilator. It is enzymatically formed **from L-arginine** and activates guanylate cyclase which increases cGMP causing **vascular smooth muscle relaxation. Answer D.**

20) Which of the following is the most prevalent anion in extracellular fluid:

a) Sodium
b) Potassium
c) Calcium
d) Chloride
e) Phosphate

See comment in the next question. **Answer D.**

21) Which of the following is the most common cation in intracellular fluid:

a) Sodium
b) Potassium
c) Calcium
d) Chloride
e) Phosphate

Cells are **negative inside** because of the pump **Na/K ATPase** that transports 2K in for every 3Na. Most common IC cation is K and EC is Na. Most common IC anion is ptn and phosphate, and most common EC anion is Cl. **Answer B.**

22) Regarding glucose metabolism, which of the following substances cannot undergo gluconeogenesis:

a) Amino acids
b) Lactic acid
c) Free fatty acids
d) Glycerol

Lipids and free fatty acids metabolism generate **acetyl CoA**, which cannot be converted to pyruvate and be used for gluconeogenesis. **Answer C.**

9

23) Which of the following cytokine is NOT responsible for increased scar formation:

a) Interferon
b) TGF-beta
c) VEGF
d) CTGF

Overexpression of growth factors, such as transforming growth factor-beta (TGF-beta), vascular endothelial growth factor (VEGF), and connective tissue growth factor (CTGF) appear to play a role in the formation of hypertrophic scars. **Answer A.**

24) Maximum collagen synthesis occurs during

a) 0-72hs
b) First 24 hours
c) 7-21 days
d) 3 weeks – 2 months

Collagen type III constitute the **early matrix** scaffolding and collagen **type I** is the **final matrix**. Around 3 weeks postinjury the amount of collagen in the wound reaches a plateau, but the **tensile strength** continues to increase for approximately **6-12 months**. **Answer C.**

2. HEMATOLOGY AND COAGULATION

1) Which type of allergic reaction is associated with Vitamin K injection:

   a) Type I
   b) Type II
   c) Type III
   d) Type IV

   Vitamin K injection has been shown to cause a delayed-type hypersensitivity reaction. Mostly after IM or SQ administration of vitamin K1, independent of the total dose. Vitamin K is necessary for the activation of the natural anticoagulants proteins C and S, and **factors II, VII, IX and X**. Deficiency presents with bleeding with **prolonged PT/INR. Answer D.**

2) What is the best test for liver synthetic function:

   a) INR
   b) PT
   c) PTT
   d) MEGX

   Aminotransferases are used to detect hepatocyte injury; **Indocyanine green** measures the **clearance capacity** of the Liver; chronic inflammation and altered immunomediation can be evaluated hepatic serologies, Immunoglobulins and autoantibodies. **Albumin and PT** are the best tests for the liver's **biosynthetic capacity**. **Answer B.**

3) What is the best test for hepatic excretory function:

a) INR
b) PT
c) PTT
d) MEGX

Monoethylglycinexylidide (**MEGX**) test, which provides a direct measure of the **actual functional state** of the liver, evaluates hepatic excretory function. MEGX is the major **Lidocaine byproduct**, which metabolism depends on the liver **cytochrome P450** system. **Answer D**.

4) Von Willebrand's disease is seen on laboratory exam to have a reliably increased:

a) Prothrombin Time
b) Antiplatelet antibodies levels
c) Ristocetin cofactor activity
d) Factor II activity

vWD is the most common congenital bleeding disorder. Patient's have long bleeding time with typical bleeding of platelet disorders. **PT is normal and PTT can be elevated** sometimes due to associated factor VIII deficiency. vWF is important for primary hemostasis by **binding platelets and endothelium**. Diagnostic tests include Plasma vWF antigen, Plasma activity (ristocetin cofactor activity) and Factor VIII activity. **Answer C.**

5) Type II von Willebrand's disease is:

a) Autosomal dominant
b) Autosomal recessive
c) Sex-linked dominant
d) Sex-linked recessive

Types I (partial deficiency) and II (qualitative defect) are autosomal dominant. Type III (total deficiency) is autosomal recessive. **Answer A.**

6) Which of the following treatment options is appropriate for all three types of von Willebrand's disease:

   a) Cryoprecipitate
   b) Conjugated estrogens
   c) DDAVP
   d) Fresh Frozen Plasma

Drug classes include desmopressin (dDAVP), vWF-containing products, antifibrinolytics, estrogens and topical thrombin. Therapy includes a trial of DDAVP in all Type I, most Type II but not in Type III. Type II has abnormal vWF itself, and therefore treatments to cause increased release of vWF, including DDAVP or estrogens, would be ineffective. **Answer A.**

7) Inheritance of Christmas disease is:

   a) Autosomal dominant
   b) Autosomal recessive
   c) X-linked dominant
   d) X-linked recessive

Hemophilia A (Factor VIII deficiency) and B, or Christmas disease (Factor IX deficiency) are X-linked recessive diseases. Lab shows **prolonged aPTT with normal platelet count and PT**. Treatment is with recombinant factor IX concentrate or FFP. Most common site of bleeding for both are into the joints. **Answer D.**

8) In Hemophilia A, levels of Factor VIII should be 100% preoperatively. Post-operatively levels should be maintained above:

a) 20%
b) 30%
c) 50%
d) 80%

Abnormal aPTT usually occurs when the levels of Factor VIII are less than 30% of the mean normal concentration. Number of units = (% x kg BW)/2 for factor VIII concentrate transfusion. **Answer B**.

9) Uremia is especially important in operative candidates because it inhibits the function of:

a) Polymorphonuclear lymphocytes
b) Macrophages
c) Platelets
d) Megakaryocytes

Uremic bleeding is caused by **impaired platelet function.** Manifestations include mucosal bleeding and easy bruising. **Answer C.**

10) Acute treatment for uremia includes:

a) Hemodialysis
b) DDAVP
c) Platelets
d) FFP

Indications for urgent hemodialysis include **fluid overload, poisoning, hyperkalemia and uremia**. Treatment options for uremic bleeding also include dDAVP, estrogens and cryoprecipitate. **Answer A.**

11) Which of the following is not an acquired thrombophilia:

    a) Inflammatory Bowel Disease
    b) Smoking
    c) Obesity
    d) Chronic Kidney disease
    e) Factor V Leiden

    IBD, smoking, obesity, CKD, chronic Liver disease, CHF, trauma, immobilization, cancer, pregnancy, drugs (Tamoxifen, HRT), OCP (most common cause of thrombosis in females) and previous thromboembolism are examples of acquired thrombofilia. **Answer E**.

12) The most common inherited hypercoagulable disorder is:

    a) Hyperhomocysteinemia
    b) Protein S deficiency
    c) Protein C deficiency
    d) Antithrombin III deficiency
    e) Factor V Leiden

    Factor Va Leiden is the most common cause of inherited thrombophilia. This factor is inactivated more slowly, increasing thrombin and coagulation. It also decreases the anticoagulant activity of **activated protein C**. Treatment usually consists of unfractionated Heparin or LMWH followed by Warfarin. Hyperhomocysteinemia can be both, inherited and acquired and a marker for atherosclerotic disease. **Answer E.**

13) Lifetime warfarin therapy is indicated in:

    a) Cancer
    b) 1st episode of DVT
    c) Recurrent idiopathic DVT
    d) Any upper extremity DVT

Recurrent idiopathic or 3rd episode of DVT are indications for lifelong Warfarin therapy. Cancer is an acquired thrombofilia and indication for therapy is until active cancer is in remission. **Answer C.**

14) Heparin's mechanism of action is:

a) Direct activation of antithrombin
b) Prevents vitamin k dependent coagulation factors
c) Direct thrombin inhibitor
d) Stimulates tPA release

Heparin is an **indirect thrombin inhibitor** which complexes with antithrombin, converting this cofactor from a slow to a rapid inactivator of thrombin, **factor Xa**, and to a lesser extent, factors XIIa, XIa, and IXa. The binding of heparin to AT accelerates the inactivation of AT 1000- to 4000-fold. **Answer A**.

15) Most common cause of death after transfusion is:

a) Disease transfusion
b) Clerical error
c) Anaphylaxis
d) TRALI

The most common cause of death is due to clerical error leading to ABO incompatibility. **Answer B**.

16) Transfusion-related acute lung injury is due to:

a) Antibodies to recipients WBCs
b) IgG reaction against IgA in IgA-deficient recipient
c) Antibodies in recipient against WBCs in donor blood
d) Reaction against plasma proteins or IgA in the transfused blood

TRALI is caused by clot in the pulmonary capillaries due to antibodies in the transfused blood against the recipients WBCs. Usually presents with respiratory distress and pulmonary infiltrates within six hours after transfusion. **Answer A.**

17) 28 year old male was brought to the emergency room after a motor vehicle accident. After initial resuscitation, FAST exam was positive for fluid in the hepatorrenal fossa. Patient received 18 units of blood and was transferred to the OR for exploratory laparotomy. Most common cause of his persistent coagulopathy is:

   a) Dilution
   b) Decreased body temperature
   c) Decreased levels of Vitamin K dependent factors
   d) Decreased calcium levels

   Calcium chelators are used for blood storage and can result in hypocalcemia following massive transfusion. Calcium is essential for the **clotting cascade**. **Answer D.**

18) Which one of the following blood products is most likely to cause bacterial contamination:

   a) Packed RBC's
   b) Fresh frozen plasma
   c) Platelets
   d) Cryoprecipitate

   Platelets have the greatest risk of infection because they are **not refrigerated**. Refrigeration also causes loss of von Willebrand factor multimers. **Gram positive bacteria** (Staph Edpidermidis and Staph Aureus) are the most common bacterial contaminants of blood products. **Answer C.**

19) Treatment for delayed hemolysis in a stable patient after transfusion of blood products is:

a) Observation
b) Fluids, diuretics, HCO3-, and vasopressors
c) Steroids
d) Invasive monitoring

Delayed hemolytic transfusion reactions are most often detected when tests reveal a positive **direct antiglobulin** test or an indirect antiglobulin test. Other findings include decreasing hemoglobin or hematocrit, and increasing indirect Bilirubin. Treatment is rarely necessary. Urine output and renal function should be monitored. **Answer A.**

20) Most common reaction to blood transfusion is:

a) Anaphylaxis
b) Febrile nonhemolytic transfusion reaction
c) Urticaria
d) TRALI

Febrile nonhemolytic transfusion reaction is the most common transfusion reaction. It requires stopping any current transfusion, supportive care, and using a **WBC filter** for any subsequent transfusions. **Answer B.**

21) Which of the following factor is the convergence point to both coagulation pathways (intrinsic and extrinsic):

a) Factor VII
b) Factor XII
c) Factor X
d) Prothrombin

Factor VII associated with tissue factor initiate the **extrinsic pathway** (evaluated by **PT** -prothrombin time). **Factor XII** and exposed collagen initiate the **intrinsic pathway** (evaluated by **PTT**). Factor X converts prothrombin (factor II) to thrombin. **Answer C.**

22) Which of the following coagulation factors has the shortest half-life:

    a) II
    b) VII
    c) VIII
    d) X

Factor **VIII** is the most **labile** factor; factors **II, VII, IX, X**, ptn C, and ptn S are **Vit K dependent** factors, and factor VII has the shortest half-life. All factors are synthesized in the endothelium, except factor VIII and vWF (liver). **Answer B.**

23) 68 year old male presents with acute retroperitoneal and lower GI bleeding POD#1 after prostatectomy. Most likely cause of his bleeding is:

    a) Prostacyclin release
    b) Protein C and S inhibition
    c) Urokinase release
    d) Fibrinogen decrease

Urokinase release can be stimulated by prostate manipulation, inducing **fibrinolysis**. Ptn C and S are physiologic anticoagulants, inhibiting factors V and VIII. **Treatment** is with **aminocaproic acid. Answer C.**

24) Which of the following factors is not evaluated by partial thromboplastin time:

   a) Factor II
   b) Factor V
   c) Factor VII
   d) Factor IX

   All of the above factors are **vitamin K dependent** (warfarin mechanism of action).PTT evaluates the intrinsic pathway but it does not measure factors VII and XIII. **Answer C.**

25) Platelet function is best evaluated by which of the following tests:

   a) Bleeding time
   b) PT/INR
   c) PTT
   d) ACT

   PT evaluates the **extrinsic pathway** and **liver synthetic function**. **PTT** evaluates the **intrinsic pathway** (**therapeutic anticoagulation** level with heparin use is between **60-90**), as does activated clotting time (routine anticoagulation level is ~200 and for cardiopulmonary bypass >400). **Answer A.**

26) An otherwise healthy 39 year old female is scheduled for elective laparoscopic cholecystectomy. Which of the following is the most appropriate DVT prophylaxis:

   a) Low molecular weight heparin
   b) Sequential compressive devices
   c) Early ambulation
   d) Subcutaneous heparin

For **low risk patients** (age < 40, no risk factors and minor procedure) DVT prevention is with **early ambulation**. Moderate to high risk patients should be managed with mechanical and pharmacological prevention. **Answer C.**

27) Post operative day 1, the same patient developed proximal thigh and leg edema. Duplex scan revealed ileofemoral deep venous thrombosis. Next step in management is:

a) LMWH 1mg/Kg BID
b) Compression stockings and leg elevation
c) Heparin drip bolus of 18u/Kg IV
d) IVC filter placement

See next comment. **Answer A.**

28) Appropriate treatment is started, but in POD#2 she presents with hematemesis and hypotension. After adequate blood transfusion and resuscitation, what is the next step in her DVT therapy:

a) Check PTT, if ≥ 60-90, hold anticoagulation
b) Stop LMWH, start heparin at 18u/kg and IVC filter placement
c) Start direct thrombin inhibitor and place IVC filter
d) IVC filter placement only

Initial treatment of lower extremity DVT is with **therapeutic anticoagulation** (LMWH at 1mg/Kg BID or **Heparin 80u/Kg bolus followed by 18u/Kg** maintenance dose). Heparin activates AT-III, it can be monitored by **PTT levels** (60-90) and reversed with **protamine. Half life** is **60-90 min**. Main indications for **IVC filter** placement include DVT or PE with complication, recurrent DVT or PE, or a **contraindication to anticoagulate. Answer D.**

29) 65 year old male was recently diagnosed with right inguinal hernia and requested you to perform a laparoscopic repair next week, during his vacation. He is currently on plavix and past history include coronary bare metal stent placement 2 months ago. Which of the following is the appropriate next step:

a) Hold plavix 5-7 days pre op and proceed with surgery
b) Reschedule the procedure and continue plavix for 1 year
c) Hold plavix, start aspirin and reschedule the procedure after 3 months
d) Hold plavix 24hs pre op, start heparin, and proceed with surgery

Regarding coronary stents, clopidogrel (plavix) should be continued for **6 weeks** if **bare metal** stents were used, and for **1 year** when **drug eluding** stents were placed. Plavix should be held 5-7 days preop, aspirin continued perioperatively, and plavix restarted postop. **Answer A.**

30) 50 year old male presents with persistent bleeding during lower extremity bypass. Heparin was given before the arteriotomy and you decide to reverse it with protamine. Which of the following is **not** a side effect of protamine use:

a) Tachycardia
b) Anaphylaxis
c) Cross-reaction with insulin
d) Hypotension

Protamine reverses heparin effects (**1mg protamine/100u Heparin**) and is associated with **hypotension**, bradicardia, and anaphylactic reaction. **Answer A.**

31) Which of the following does not occur during red blood cell storage:

   a) Potassium increase
   b) pH level decrease
   c) 2.3 DPG increase
   d) Lactic acid increase
   e) Calcium decrease

   PRBCs should not be stored longer than 3 weeks. **Massive transfusion** can lead to **hypocalcemia** because of the preservation solution (**citrate binds calcium**).2.3 DPG, potassium, and lactic acid levels increase. **Answer C.**

32) 32 year old male presented with fever and acute onset respiratory distress 4 hours after blood transfusion. Which of the following is false regarding transfusion related acute lung injury:

   a) Occurs in less than 24hs after blood transfusion
   b) Pulmonary wedge pressure are < 18mmHg
   c) Caused by donor antibodies against recipient WBC's
   d) More common than hemolytic transfusion reaction

   TRALI is a **non cardiogenic pulmonary edema** caused by donor anibodies against recipient WBC's. Usually occurs **less than 6hs** after transfusion. Symptoms are **similar to ARDS**, and consists of fever, hypoxia, and diffuse alveolar infiltrates. **Answer A.**

33) Regarding Vitamin K, which of the following is true:

   a) Antagonized by heparin
   b) Synthesized by GI flora
   c) Binds to thrombin to facilitate coagulation
   d) Normalizes PTT in liver failure

Vitamin K is **fat soluble** and essential for activity of several carboxylase enzymes within the hepatic cells, and is necessary for the **activation of coagulation factors** II, VII, IX, and X. **Proteins C and S** also require vitamin K for their activity. Dietary vitamin K1 is found in green vegetables and gut flora synthesizes vitamin K2. **Deficiency** manifests as **prolonged PT and INR. Answer B.**

3. TRANSPLANT IMMUNOLOGY AND SURGICAL ONCOLOGY

1) The Major Histocompatibility Complex known as HLA is coded by a series of genes located on which chromosome:

   a) 2
   b) 4
   c) 6
   d) 8

   Located on chromosome 6 in humans, the function of MHC molecules is to **bind peptide fragments derived from pathogens and display them on the cell surface** for recognition by the appropriate T cells. As a result, virus-infected cells are killed, macrophages are activated, and B cells are stimulated to produce antibodies. **Answer C.**

2) What percentage of nucleated cells has Class I molecules:

   a) 20%
   b) 50%
   c) 80%
   d) 100%

   Class I MHC molecules are expressed on all nucleated cells. Class II MHC molecules are expressed by antigen presenting cells. **Answer D**.

3) All of the following are classified as antigen presenting cells, except:

   a) B lymphocytes
   b) Monocytes
   c) Dendritic cells
   d) Platelets

APCs include dendritic cells, macrophages, and B-lymphocytes. They express both MHC-I and MHC-II molecules and serve two major functions during adaptive immunity: antigens processing for presentation to T-lymphocytes, and stimulate differentiation of lymphocytes. Platelets are not considered an antigen-presenting cell. Rather, they play a role in primary hemostasis forming platelet plug. **Answer D.**

4) The main responsible for chronic and subacute rejection is:

   a) B cell
   b) Natural killer cells
   c) T cell
   d) Dendritic cells

Diagnosis is usually based on histological signs such as infiltrating T cells, accompanied by eosinophils, plasma cells, and neutrophils , compromise of tissue anatomy, and injury to blood vessels. T cells, stimulated by IL-2, causes proliferation and differentiation of itself. **Answer C.**

5) Prevention of hyperacute rejection is best done by:

   a) ABO compatibility testing
   b) In vitro studies
   c) Cross-match studies
   d) All of the above

Hyperacute rejection usually occurs within minutes due to the presence of preformed antibodies. You can prevent this by **ABO compatibility testing** and cross-match studies (in vitro). **Answer A.**

6) 23-year-old male status post a kidney transplant is found to have graft rejection within days of receiving his transplant. Biopsy would show:

a) Atrophy and fibrosis
b) Cellular infiltrate, membrane damage, and apoptosis
c) Accumulation of mast cells
d) Tubulitis and endarteritis

Through modern day immunosuppression, acute rejection is not as common as before. When experienced, biopsy will reveal **primarily lymphocytic infiltrates**, and signs of apoptosis. **Answer B**.

7) 35 years old female on immunosuppressive regimen involving corticosteroids. Typical adverse effects include all of the following, except:

a) Septic joint necrosis
b) Pancreatitis
c) Lipodystrophy
d) Growth supression

Classic effects of **corticosteroids** include glucose intolerance, breakdown of muscle, redistribution of fat, the well-known Wickham's striae, electrolyte abnormalities, hypertension, hyperglycemia, pancreatitis, hematologic, immunologic, and neuropsychologic effects. **Long-term** use may be associated with **osteoporosis**, aseptic joint necrosis, adrenal insufficiency, GI and Liver effects, hyperlipidemia, growth suppression, and possible congenital malformations. **Answer A.**

8) Azathioprine mechanism of action consists of:

a) Stops the signal IL-2
b) Inhibiting calcineurin
c) Is a antimetabolite
d) Binds to cyclophilin

Azathioprine is effective in preventing immune rejection. It does this by preventing **DNA and RNA synthesis**, thus prohibiting the synthesis of B and T lymphocytes.
Answer C.

9) The most common malignancies in transplanted patients is (are):

a) Skin cancers
b) Lymphoma
c) Leukemia
d) Hepatocellular

Following **solid organ transplantation**, recipients have a **higher incidence of skin cancers** (mostly SCC) but also BCC, melanomas, and Merkel cell cancers; non-Hodgkin's and Hodgkin lymphoma, Kaposi's sarcoma, cervical CA, RCC, HCC, and a variety of sarcomas. A 20-fold increase in nonmelanoma skin cancers, Kaposi's sarcoma, and non-Hodgkin lymphomas was noted. **Answer A.**

10) Regarding donor and recipient matching, which of the following is the most important antigen:

a) HLA - A
b) HLA - DP
c) HLA - DQ
d) HLA - DR

Human leukocyte antigen (**HLA**), is considered the main responsible for acute and chronic **rejection**. **Class I** includes HLA – A, HLA-B, and HLA-C. **Class II** includes HLA-DP, HLA-DQ, and HLA-DR (most important).
Answer D.

11) Which of the following transplant procedures does not require a preoperative crossmatch:

a) Heart
b) Lung
c) Liver
d) Kidney

A crossmatch reaction identifies **preformed antibodies** in the recipient serum after mixing it with the donor lymphocytes. Most heart and lung and all pancreas and kidney need preoperative crossmatch. **Answer C.**

12) 51 year old male, history of renal transplant last year and complicated laparoscopic cholecystectomy 2 weeeks ago, presents with elevated creatinine and anuria. During his cholecystectomy, a hepatic duct injury was identified and a T-tube drain was left in place. Which of the following is most likely being used for his immunosuppressive therapy:

a) Mycophenolate
b) Cyclosporin
c) Azathioprine
d) Tacrolimus

Cyclosporin **inhibits** cytokine synthesis, mainly **IL-2 and IL-4** and it undergoes **enterohepatic re-circulation**. Bile drainage may decrease this drug levels and cause rejection. Side effects include **nephro and hepatotoxicity**.
Answer B.

13) A 60 year old male was placed on the waiting list for renal transplant. His twin brother is willing to donate one of his kidneys. Which of the following is not considered a contraindication for living kidney donors:

a) Hepatitis B
b) Hepatitis C
c) Diabetes Mellitus
d) Dual collecting systems

Viral infections, such as HIV and **hepatitis** B/C, cocaine use, **DM**, simultaneous cancer or infection and severe cardiopulmonary disease are all **contraindications** for living kidney donation. Most common **cause of death in donors** is **pulmonary embolism. Answer D.**

14) Regarding liver transplantation, which of the following is the most common indication:

a) Chronic Hepatitis B
b) Chronic Hepatitis C
c) Hepatocellular carcinoma
d) Primary Sclerosing cholangitis

In **children**, the most common indication is **biliary atresia. Contraindications** for liver transplant include severe cardiopulmonary disease, active **ETOH abuse**, infection, or cancer elsewhere. **Answer B.**

15) Which of the following is **not** a contraindication for liver transplantation:

a) Portal Vein Thrombosis
b) Urosepsis
c) Cholangiocarcinoma
d) Active ulcerative colitis

If certain criteria is met (**Milan criteria**), patients with **HCC** can still undergo transplantation. Those include single **tumor < 5cm or 3 lesions < 3cm each**. Age and portal vein thrombosis are also not contraindications. **Answer A.**

4. SURGICAL INFECTIONS AND ANTIBIOTICS

1) Which of the following is **not** part of the systemic inflammatory response syndrome criteria:

a) Temperature < 36C or > 38.3C
b) Hear rate > 90 BPMs
c) Respiratory rate > 20/min
d) AST > 250
e) WBC >12,000 or < 4,000

SIRS is the clinical syndrome that results from a dysregulated inflammatory response to a **noninfectious insult**, such as pancreatitis, burns, or surgery. It requires that two or more of the above criterias be present. Although AST is a marker for a generalized inflammatory process and liver failure, it is not part of the clinical diagnosis of SIRS. It is used in Ranson's criteria. **Answer D.**

2) Catalase is an enzyme responsible for metabolizing:

a) Reactive oxygen species
b) Free hydrogen ions in an excessively acidic environment
c) Beta lactam antibiotics
d) Protein degradation biproducts

Reactive oxygen species are metabolized by catalase, absent in anaerobic bacteria. **Answer A.**

3) Empiric antimicrobial therapy comprises:

a) A single dose of antibiotic required
b) Discontinuing therapy within 24 hours according to SCIP criteria
c) Use of agents for 3-5 days when risk of surgical infection is high
d) Treatment until cultures return

Empiric therapy uses an antimicrobial agent based on the suspected source of infection and the most likely organisms. **Answer D.**

4) Linezolid mechanism of action affects:

   a) Cell wall synthesis
   b) 50S ribosomal activity
   c) Folate metabolism
   d) 30S ribosomal activity

   Linezolid is a oxazolidinone that works by inhibiting the 50S ribosomal subunit, inhibiting bacterial protein synthesis (**bacteriostatic**). It has activity against **gram positive** organisms including VRE, MSSA, and MRSA. **Answer B**.

5) Trimethoprim-sulfamethoxazole mechanism of action affects:

   a) Cell wall synthesis
   b) 50S ribosomal activity
   c) Folate metabolism
   d) 30S ribosomal activity

   TMP-SMX works by inhibiting sequential steps of **folate synthesis** (bactericidal). It has reliable activity against aerobic **gram positive and gram negative** bacteria, including MSSA and E Coli. Resistance is based upon decreased permeability or a target enzyme with decreased affinity for the drugs. **Answer C.**

6) Tobramycin mechanism of action affects :

   a) Cell wall synthesis
   b) 50S ribosomal activity
   c) Folate metabolism
   d) 30S ribosomal activity

Aminoglycosides work by alteration of the cell membrane and binding to the 30S ribosomal subunit, leading to misreading of the genetic code and inhibition of translocation. **Bactericidal** against aerobic **gram negatives**, including Enterobacteriaceae, Pseudomonas, and Haemophilus influenzae. **Answer D**.

7) Cephalosporins mechanism of action affect:

   a) Cell wall synthesis
   b) 50S ribosomal activity
   c) Folate metabolism
   d) 30S ribosomal activity

Beta-lactam antibiotics are generally **bactericidal** and the mechanism of action is an indirect inhibition of bacterial **cell wall synthesis**, binding to penicillin-binding protein. Bacterial resistance is by decreased penetration to the target site, alteration of the target site, and inactivation of the antibiotic by a bacterial enzyme. **Answer A**.

8) Infection risk for class I clean wound is:

   a) 0 - 2.0%
   b) 1.0 - 3.0%
   c) 4.0 - 8.0%
   d) 6.0 - 10.0%

Clean wounds, such as hernia repair or breast biopsies, have an expected infection rate of approximately 1.0-3.0%. **Answer B**.

9) Infection risk for class II clean/contaminated wound is:

   a) 1.0 - 5.0%
   b) 2.0 - 8.0%
   c) 3.0 - 13.0%
   d) 3.0 - 10.0%

Clean-contaminated wounds include those with a **hollow viscus** such as respiratory, alimentary, or genitourinary tracts that is opened **under controlled circumstances**. **Answer B.**

10) Infection risk for class III contaminated wound is:

   a) 1.0-6.0%
   b) 2.0-8.0%
   c) 3.0- 9.0%
   d) 6.0-15.0%

Contaminated wounds are open accidental wounds encountered early after injury, those with **extensive introduction of bacteria** into a normally sterile are of the body due to **major breaks in sterile technique**, gross spillage of viscous contents. **Answer D**.

11) Infection risk for class IV dirty wound is:

   a) 1.0 - 5.0%
   b) 9.0 - 18.0%
   c) 6.0 - 20.0%
   d) 7.0 - 30.0%

Dirty wounds are wounds with high degree of contamination, such as perforated appendicitis and gunshot wound to the colon. **Answer D.**

12) A 55 year old female presents with left lower quadrant abdominal pain. CT scan of the abdomen and pelvis showed a 5cm x 6cm abscess and thickened sigmoid colon. Best treatment is:

   a) NPO, IV antibiotics
   b) Broad spectrum PO antibiotics
   c) IV antibiotics and CT guided drainage
   d) Hartmann's Procedure

Complicated diverticulitis (with abscess, obstruction or fistula) as in this case, should be managed with hospital admission, bowel rest, IV antibiotics and percutaneous drainage of the abscess if possible. Uncomplicated cases can be managed as outpatient with PO antibiotics. **Answer C**.

13)   Fluoroquinolones mechanism of action affect :

a) Cell wall synthesis
b) Topoisomerase
c) Folate metabolism
d) 30S ribosomal activity

Quinolones are **bactericidal** and inhibit Topoisomerase II and IV, interfering with **DNA synthesis**. **Answer B**.

14)   The main reason of administering a prophylactic, single dose cephalosporin in elective colorectal surgery is to :

a) Prevent intra abdominal abscess formation
b) Prevent anastomotic leak
c) Prevent wound infection
d) Prevent urinary tract infection

The single dose preoperative antibiotic prophylaxis is used to prevent surgical site infections and has the **same results as multiple pre and post operative doses**. **Answer C**.

15)   Which of the following is the most common infection in surgical patients:

a) Pneumonia
b) UTI
c) Wound Infection
d) Colitis

Most common infection in **medical patients is UTI**. SSIs are the most common (35%) nosocomial infection among surgical patients. **Answer C**.

16) 61 year old female is admitted to SICU with ascending cholangitis, and 24hs later develops hypotension and mental status change. Which of the following is expected during this phase of septic shock:

a) Increased Insulin; Increased Glucose
b) Increased Insulin; Decreased Glucose
c) Decreased Insulin; Decreased Glucose
d) Decreased Insulin; Increased Glucose

Early sepsis is shown to have increased glucose and decreased insulin because of **impaired glucose utilization**. **Late sepsis** will present with increased glucose and insulin levels because of increased **insulin resistance. Answer D**.

17) 71 year old male with complicated diverticulitis had an exploratory laparotomy with left hemicolectomy. Few days later he developed a wound infection and culture is taken. What is the most common anaerobe found in surgical site infections:

a) Escherichia coli
b) Staphilococcus epidermidis
c) Bacteriodes fragilis
d) Clostridium Perfringens

B. fragilis is the **most common anaerobe** that is found in surgical wound infections and the most common anaerobe found in the colon. **E.coli** is the most common **Gram negative rod** found in surgical wound infections. **Answer C**.

18) A chronic renal patient is unable to use her AV fistula for hemodialysis. A dialysis catheter is placed and 5 days later she presents with fever, chills, and elevated WBC. What is the most likely organism causing her symptoms:

    a) Staph epidermidis
    b) Staph aureus
    c) Escherichia coli
    d) C. albicans

    Coagulase-negative staphylococci are a common constituent of the **skin flora** and have surpassed S. aureus as the major cause of central venous catheters -related bloodstream infection. The deposition of **biofilm** on the surface of CVC is thought to play an important role in the colonization process. **Gram-negative bacilli** (K. Pneumoniae) account for up to **1/3**, and **Fungi** (Candida species), account for up to 20% of **systemic infections** associated with CVCs. **Answer A**.

19) A patient with HIV comes to the ER complaining of severe right lower quadrant pain associated with fever, nausea and diarrhea for the past 48hs. Lab results are significant for elevated WBC. Patient had an emergency laparotomy. What is the most common infectious cause of his acute surgical intervention:

    a) CMV
    b) Salmonella
    c) Cryptococcus
    d) Yersinia entericolitica

Opportunistic infections with bacteria (Salmonella), fungi (Cryptococcus), protozoa
(Toxoplasmosis, Cryptosporidiosis), and viruses (CMV) can cause several **GI symptoms**, especially **diarrhea. CMV** may cause **severe enterocolitis** and is the most common infectious cause of emergency laparotomy. C. difficile is a major concern in patients who were recently on antibiotics. **Answer B**.

20) Which of the following options describes the mechanism of Vancomycin resistance by Enterococci:

   a) Mutation in the cell-wall binding protein
   b) Plasmid with antibiotic resistance
   c) Decrease in active transport
   d) Mutation in DNA gyrase

   Vancomycin is restricted to **gram-positive** bacteria and it is the **first choice for MRSA** and S. epidermidis infection therapy. It is also an **alternative** agent **for enterococcal** infection as ampicillin resistance continues to increase. Resistance is associated with synthesis of a plasmid-encoded ligase that results in synthesis of cell wall precursors that will not bind vancomycin. **Answer A.**

21) Which of the following options describes the mechanism of penicillin resistance:

   a) Mutation in the cell-wall binding protein
   b) Plasmid with antibiotic resistance
   c) Decrease in active transport
   d) Mutation in DNA gyrase

   The antibacterial effect of penicillins involves **binding to** penicillin binding proteins (**PBPs**) in the cell wall of susceptible bacteria. **Hydrolysis of the Beta-lactam bond by Beta-lactamase** is the most important mechanism of bacterial resistance to penicillins. **Answer B**.

22) Which of the following options describes the mechanism of gentamicin resistance:

a) By a mutation in the cell-wall binding protein
b) By a plasmid with antibiotic resistance
c) By a decrease in active transport
d) By a mutation in DNA gyrase

There are two major mechanisms by which resistance of gram-negative organisms to aminoglycosides occur: Bacterial production of **inactivating enzymes** and **decreased accumulation** of the drug by an efflux system. **Answer C**.

23) Which of the following options describes the mechanism by which Staph aureus become Methicillin-resistant:

a) Mutation in the cell-wall binding protein
b) Plasmid with antibiotic resistance
c) Decrease in active transport
d) Mutation in DNA gyrase

Like vancomycin resistance, Methicillin resistance is acquired by a mutation in the cell-wall binding protein. Mutation in **DNA gyrase** is associated with resistance to **Quinolones**. **Answer A**.

24) Which of the following aminoacids is the most abundant in the body:

a) Leucine
b) Isoleucine
c) Valine
d) Glutamine

Glutamine is the most abundant **nonessential amino acid** in the human body. It is considered as a **primary fuel for enterocytes, macrophages,** and **limphocytes**. It accounts for a major portion of the AA released by muscle during catabolic states and has been used in short gut syndrome. Leucine, valine and isoleucine are essential amino acids . **Answer D.**

25) A 52-year-old female with Barret's esophagus and high grade dysplasia, requires nutritional supplementation with TPN for three days. Which of the following elements are not necessary in her TPN solution:

a) Chromium
b) Copper
c) Iron
d) Zinc

Short term TPN **does not require iron or iodine**. Most hospitalized patients who will need TPN for less than one to two weeks fall within this scope. Patients who require prolonged TPN will require this supplementation. All TPN mixtures include zinc, copper, chromium, and selenium. **Answer C.**

26) 65 year old male, diabetic, allergic to Penicillin, develops left foot gangrene after hitting his toe. Cultures revealed clostridium perfringens. Antibiotic of choice is:

a) Metronidazol
b) Vancomycin
c) Gentamicin
d) Clindamycin

Antibiotics are often essential but are ineffective without **primary surgical intervention. Broad empiric regimens** include penicillin with aminoglycoside. Clindamycin can be used in combination with penicillin or in allergic patients. Imipenem is a second option. **Answer D.**

27) 27 year old African American male presents with left toe osteomyelitis. Patient was diagnosed with sickle cell disease during childhood. Most common responsible bacteria is:

a) Haemophilus influenza
b) Staphylococcus aureus
c) Streptococcus species
d) Salmonella species

Even though **Salmonella** species are **frequently encountered**, they rarely cause bone infection. *Staphylococcus aureus* is the most common organism in sickle cell osteomyelitis episodes. **Answer B.**

28) Which of the following organisms produce exotoxin as a virulence mechanism:

a) Pseudomonas
b) Streptococcus
c) Klebsiella
d) E. Coli

Gram negative and Gram positive bacteria produce endotoxin and exotoxin respectively. Gram positive bacteria have several virulence mechanisms, including streptolysin , pyrogenic exotoxins, M-ptn and the cell wall. **Answer B.**

5. PHARMACOLOGY AND ANESTHESIA

1) Tardive dyskinesia is a side effect of medical therapy, treatment includes:

   a) Haloperidol
   b) Diphendydramine
   c) Promethazine
   d) Propanolol

   TD is a hyperkinetic movement disorder that appears after **prolonged use of dopamine receptor blocking agents**, mainly antipsychotic drugs and the antiemetic drug, metoclopramide. **Diphenhydramine and benztropine** have been shown to lower rates of tardive dyskinesia if taken with antipsychotic medications. **Answer B**.

2) Inducers of Cytochrome P450 (CYP) include:

   a) Cholestyramine
   b) Niacin
   c) MAOIs
   d) ETOH

   CYP enzymes are present in most tissues of the body, and play important roles in hormone **synthesis and breakdown**. They also function in **toxic compounds metabolism** (drugs), and endogenous metabolism such as bilirubin, mostly in the liver. Potent inducers include: Phenytoin, Warfarin, Barbiturates, Rifampicin, Carbamazepine, ETOH, Dilantin, and smoking. **Answer D**.

3) Inhibitors of Cytochrome P450 (CYP) include:

a) Flagyl
b) Insecticides
c) Adenosine
d) Metoclopramide

Potent inhibitors include: Erythromycin, Fluconazole, Flagyl, Cimetidine, Ciprofloxacin and Amiodarone. **Answer A.**

4) Efficacy is defined as:

a) Ability to achieve result without untoward effect
b) Tolerance after only a few doses
c) Effect at an unusually low dose
d) Dose required for effect

Efficacy is the ability of a drug to achieve result without untoward effects. It indicates the **capacity for a therapeutic effect** of a specific intervention. **Answer A**.

5) Tachyphylaxis is:

a) Ability to achieve result without untoward effect
b) Tolerance after only a few doses
c) Effect at an unusually low dose
d) Dose required for effect

Tachyphylaxis is a **fast response** to a medication in which the patient has **tolerance after just a few doses**. **Answer B.**

6) Which of the following drug is stored in the bones:

a) Sulfonamides
b) Ciprofloxacin
c) Ketoconazole
d) Tetracycline

Heavy metals, fluoride and tetracycline are stored in bones.
Answer D.

7) In a patient with colonic pseudobstruction, neostigmine is often used as a first line therapy. Which drug is used to counteract neostigmine's main side effect:

a) Adenosine
b) Atropine
c) Beta-blockers
d) Epinephrine

Neostigmine is an acetylcholinesterase inhibitor and the standard dose in adults is 2.0 mg IV with cardiovascular monitoring. Side effects include **bronchospasm, hypotension, abdominal pain, salivation and vomiting**. Symptomatic bradycardia causing cardiac arrest requiring atropine is also described. Atropine is a nonselective competitive antagonist for muscarinic acetylcholine receptors. **Answer B.**

8) Minimum alveolar concentration is inversely proportional to potency via lipid solubility. Which of the following is the fastest inhalational induction agent:

a) Nitrous Oxide
b) Sevoflurane
c) Isofluorane
d) Desoflurane

MAC represents the percent or concentration of a gas that causes 50% of patients to become unresponsive to a surgical stimulus. Nitrous oxide is the inhalation agent with the **highest MAC** (the least potent anesthetic gas), therefore lowest lipid solubility and **fastest onset of action**.
Answer A.

9) All of the following are true regarding Propofol, **except**:

   a) It should not be used in patients with egg allergy
   b) Metabolized in liver
   c) Causes some hypotension and respiratory depression
   d) Provides analgesia and sedation

   Propofol is used for induction and maintenance of
   anesthesia. Advantages include **rapid recovery** whereas
   disadvantages include a high incidence of **apnea**, and
   hypotension. Mechanism of action is through potentiation
   of GABA receptor activity. Metabolized in the liver,
   propofol has **no analgesic properties**. **Answer D.**

10) 45 year old male, history of ETOH abuse was admitted
    after MVA followed by rapid sequence intubation for
    airway protection. 24hs he presented with refractory
    hypotension. FAST exam, Pelvic X-Ray and CXR were
    negative. Most likely diagnosis is:

    a) Adrenocortical suppression
    b) Hyponatremia
    c) ETOH withdrawal
    d) Propofol Infusion Syndrome

    RSI involves administration of an induction agent (eg,
    etomidate) followed by a paralytic agent (eg, succinylcholine,
    rocuronium) to render the patient unconscious and
    paralyzed within 1 minute. Etomidate is a reversible
    inhibitor of 11-beta-hydroxylase, which converts 11-
    deoxycortisol to cortisol. It is the **most hemodynamically
    neutral** of the sedatives used for RSI, provides **no
    analgesia**, and side-effects include **adrenal suppression**,
    myoclonus, and evidence of cerebral excitation. **Answer A.**

11) Nondepolarizing agents can be reversed with:

   a) Edrophonium
   b) Succinylcholine
   c) Atropine
   d) Narcan

   Edrophonium and neostigmine are both
   acetylcholinesterase inhibitors, and therefore would
   increase the Acetylcholine available to compete at the
   neuromuscular junction. **Answer A.**

12) Infected areas are difficult to anesthetize secondary to:

   a) Bacterial byproducts
   b) Edema
   c) Local acidosis
   d) Incomplete injection into subdermal tissue

   All local anesthetic agents are weak bases. Infected tissue
   tends to be a more acidic environment than usual. With
   decreased PH, the fraction of unionised local anesthetic is
   decreased and consequently the **effect is reduced**.
   Answer C.

13) Epinephrine is mixed into local anesthetic in order to:

   a) Decrease bleeding
   b) Allow higher doses to be used
   c) Epinephrine also provides some anesthesia
   d) Epinephrine works directly on local nerves to excite Na
      channels to respond to amide anesthetics

   Constriction of arterioles and venules, although may prevent
   some bleeding not otherwise seen, allows less to be
   absorbed systemically. Therefore more can be injected
   locally without systemic side effects. **Answer B.**

14) Lidocaine toxicity usually presents first with:

   a) Peri-oral numbness
   b) Seizures
   c) Hypotension
   d) Tachycardia

   Lidocaine is an amide local anesthetic with mechanism of
   action at the nerve axon sodium channels. Lidocaine
   toxicity may be observed at 6 mcg/mL, and because of its
   hepatic metabolism, patients with liver dysfunction are at
   increased risk. Earlier manifestations are due to **CNS
   excitation, followed by cardiovascular changes**.
   Answer A.

15) 15 year old male remained intubated in SICU after MVA.
   Work up revealed femur fracture, Grade III splenic injury
   and duodenal hematoma. Patient had daily NGT output of
   1L, was on parenteral nutrition, intubated and sedated with
   propofol.48hs after admission, patient presented refractory
   bradycardia, base deficit 20mmol/l and myoglobinuria.
   Most likely diagnosis is:

   a) Hypocloremic metabolic alkalosis from NGT output
   b) Acute liver failure
   c) Propofol infusion syndrome
   d) Copper deficiency

   The main features of PRIS consist of **cardiac failure,
   rhabdomyolysis, severe metabolic acidosis** (base deficit
   > 10 mmol.l), **hyperlipidemia, fatty liver, and renal
   failure**. Usually occurs in young patients at doses higher
   than 5 mg/kg/h for more than 48 h. **Answer C.**

16) A 61 year old female is POD#1 after elective surgery with spinal anesthesia. She is complaining of tinnitus and recurrent headache that worsens when she tries to stand up. Initial management include all of the following, **except**:

   a) Blood patch
   b) Caffeine administration
   c) Analgesics
   d) Increase fluid intake

   Initial treatment of **post spinal anesthesia headache** is **conservative** and usually consists of bed rest, fluids, analgesics, and caffeine administration. **Blood patch** is also an option, but **more invasive** and used when other treatments fail. Symptoms include worsening headache when moving from sitting to standing position, tinnitus, diplopia, and decreased hearing. **Answer A.**

17) Which of the following options has the correct maximum anesthetic doses :

   a) Bupivacaine with epinephrine : 2.5mg/Kg
   b) Bupivacaine : 2.5mg/Kg
   c) Lidocaine: 7 mg/Kg
   d) Lidocaine with epinephrine: 5 mg/Kg

   Correct maximum anesthetic doses are: Bupivacaine: 2.5mg/K ; Lidocaine: 5 mg/Kg; and Lidocaine with epinephrine: 7 mg/Kg. **Answer B.**

6. SURGICAL NUTRITION

1) What is the average nutritional need for a healthy adult:

   a) 15 kcal/kg/day
   b) 25 kcal/kg/day
   c) 35 kcal/kg/day
   d) 50 kcal/kg/day

   A goal of 25 to 30 kcal/kg per day is reasonable for most stable patients. A goal of 35 kcal/kg per day is acceptable if weight gain is desired. This can double in hypermetabolic states. **Answer B.**

2) What is the average daily protein need for a healthy adult:

   a) 1g/kg/day
   b) 5 g/kg/day
   c) 10 g/kg/day
   d) 15 g/kg/day

   Patients with mild to moderate diseases require an average of 1g/kg per day. Critically ill patients generally require up to 1.5 g/kg per day and patients with severe burns may need as much as 2.0 g/kg per day. **Answer A.**

3) What is the increased caloric needs of a woman who is lactating:

   a) 300 kcal/day
   b) 500 kcal/day
   c) 700 kcal/day
   d) 900 kcal/day

   The average lactating woman needs an additional 500 kcal/day. **Answer B.**

4) What is the half life of albumin:

a) 1 week
b) 2 weeks
c) 3 weeks
d) 4 weeks

Hypoalbuminemia is a relatively late manifestation of malnutrition, since albumin has a half-life of **21 days** and hepatic synthetic reserve is very large. Mortality is higher in patients with a concentration < 3 g/dL. **Transferrin** has a half life of **10 days** and **prealbumin** of **2 days**. **Answer C.**

5) Which of the following is not an obligate glucose user:

a) Peripheral nerves
b) Adrenal medulla
c) Red blood cells
d) Myocytes

Glucose homeostasis is essential because certain tissues, such as **brain, erythrocytes, and cells of the renal medulla** are obligate glucose users. During starvation the body must have gluconeogenesis for those tissues. Myocytes can use multiple sources of fuel. **Answer D.**

6) Cachexia is mediated by which of the following cytokines:

a) TNF-alpha
b) Interferon gamma
c) IL-10
d) IL-6

TNF alpha mediates cachexia, Interferon gamma has multiple functions including inhibition of viral replication. **IL 10 is anti-inflammatory** and IL-6 is proinflammatory. **Answer A.**

7) 65 year old male is on post operative day 15 after sigmoid colectomy for perforated diverticulitis. Due to poor nutritional status, patient was placed on TPN and now presents with wound dehiscence, hair loss and non specific rash. Which of the following is the most likely vitamin deficiency:

a) Zinc
b) Copper
c) Selenium
d) Chromium

Copper deficiency causes **pancytopenia, selenium** deficiency leads to **cardiomyopathy, weakness, and hair loss** and **chromium** deficiency causes **hyperglycemia**, encephalopathy, and neuropathy. **Answer A.**

8) Which vitamin deficiency causes night blindness:

a) Vitamin A
b) Vitamin K
c) Vitamin D
d) Vitamin E

Vitamin K deficiency causes coagulopathy, vitamin D deficiency causes rickets and osteomalacia and vitamin E deficiency causes neuropathy. **Answer A.**

9) During the first week of starvation, which of the following is true:

a) Brain metabolism depends on protein breakdown
b) Calories are mainly supplied by fat breakdown
c) Insulin levels decrease
d) Carbohydrate reserve is depleted in the first 72hs

The blood-glucose level begins to drop several hours after a meal, leading to a decrease in insulin secretion and a rise in glucagon secretion. After one week, **muscle and liver use fatty acids** as fuel and the **brain adapts to use ketone** for metabolism. Carbohydrate reserve is depleted by 24hs. **Answer B.**

10) 65 year old male on post operative day 5 after subtotal gastrectomy is receiving parenteral nutrition. After reviewing the TPN order you noticed that the he is receiving an excess of carbohydrate. Which of the following is the expected R/Q ratio for this patient:

   a) 1.0
   b) 0.8
   c) < 0.7
   d) >1.0

   RQ is the volume of CO_2 (VCO2) produced divided by the volume of oxygen consumed (VO2). Patients utilizing 100% carbohydrate for energy, R/Q = 1.0. For **fats, R/Q ~ 0.7**. On a **mixed diet, R/Q at rest is 0.82** and for a **starving** individual, **R/Q may be as low as 0.7**. **Answer D.**

11) What is the primary fuel source for small bowel:

   a) Fatty acids
   b) Glutamine
   c) Alanine
   d) Protein

   Glutamine is the most abundant amino acid in the body and is the major fuel source of **Cancer cells and enterocytes**, being essential for the maintenance of intestinal mucosal integrity and function. It also maintains immune function by serving as the principle metabolic fuel for lymphocytes and macrophages. **Short chain fatty** acids are the primary fuel source for the **colon. Answer B.**

12) A 40 year old female comes to the emergency room with a laceration on her left arm. She is taking prednisone for severe COPD. In addition to primary closure of her wound what recommendations would you make:

a) Stop Prednisone
b) Taper Prednisone
c) Give Vitamin A
d) Give Vitamin C

Vitamin A has been shown to increase collagen synthesis and **improve wound healing** in patients on **steroids**. **Answer C.**

13) How many kcal/g does a solution with 50g dextrose, 100g of fat and 20g of protein contain:

a) 1180
b) 1150
c) 1250
d) 650

Dextrose contains 3.4 kcal/g. Protein and carbohydrates contain 4 and fat contains 9. **Answer B.**

14) Which of the following electrolyte abnormalities is not commonly seen in Refeeding syndrome:

a) Hypokalemia
b) Hypomagnesemia
c) Hypophosphatemia
d) Hyponatremia

Refeeding syndrome occurs when previously **malnourished patients** are fed with high carbohydrate loads, the result is a **rapid fall in phosphate, magnesium and potassium**, along with an increasing ECF volume. Serum phosphate concentrations of less than 0.50 mmol/l can produce the clinical features, which include impaired glucose utilization, rhabdomyolysis, leucocyte dysfunction, **respiratory and cardiac failure**, hypotension, arrhythmias, seizures, coma, and death. **Answer D**.

15) Which of the following is not a common complication of long term parenteral feeding:

   a) Hypoglycemia
   b) Intestinal Atrophy
   c) Gallstones
   d) Sepsis

   Complications of TPN fall into two main categories: I) **Catheter-related** and II) **Metabolic**. Long term TPN is associated with sepsis (from catheter colonization), hyperglycemia (from glucose impaired utilization), cholestasis and liver steatosis. **Answer A**.

16) A 21 year old college student was having a good old fashion barbecue when he squirted lighter fluid on the flames and was burned over 40% of his body. After being fluid resuscitated in the Emergency Department, the patient was transferred to the ICU. Weight of the patient on admission was 75 kg. Which of the following is his adequate caloric need:

   a) 1875 kcal/day
   b) 2200 kcal/day
   c) 1887 kcal/day
   d) 1500 kcal/day

Caloric need for a burn patient: 25 kcal/kg/day + (**30 kcal x % burned**) 25 kcal x 75 kg = 1875 + (30 kcal x .4) = 1887 kcal/day. **Answer C.**

17) The patient above was intubated due to upper airway edema following the accident. A post pyloric tube was placed and you are tasked with calculating the patient's protein needs, that are:

    a) 76 gm/day
    b) 75 gm/day
    c) 65 gm/day
    d) 82 gm/day

    Protein oxidation rates are approximately 50% greater in burn patients than in normal patients. Protein need for a burn patient: **1gm/kg/day + (3gm x % burned)** 1 gm x 75 kg = 75 + (3 gm x .4) = 76 gm/day. **Answer A.**

18) A 76 year old male is admitted to the hospital with weakness, fatigue and a 22 pound unintended weight loss over the last 6 months. On abdominal exam, a mass is palpated in the patient's right lower quadrant. A CT of the abdomen and pelvis confirms a 6 x 7 cm mass in the ascending colon. The tumor is resected and pathology confirms adenocarcinoma. Which of the following acts as a primary fuel source for neoplastic cells:

    a) Medium-chain fatty acids
    b) Long-chain fatty acids
    c) Short-chain fatty acids
    d) Glutamine

    Glutamine can act as fuel for **neoplastic cells** as well as for small bowel **enterocytes**. Glutamine is the most common amino acid in the bloodstream and the tissues and can be used as a substrate for **gluconeogenesis**. **Short-chain fatty acids** can act as fuel for **colonocytes**. **Answer D.**

19) The above patient described a 11 Kg unintended weight loss over the last 6 months. Which of the following indicators of his nutritional status is the strongest risk factor for post-operative morbidity and mortality:

a) Total lymphocyte count
b) Transferrin
c) Prealbumin
d) Retinal binding protein
e) Albumin

Albumin (half life 20 days) ≤ than 3 is the strongest risk factor of post-op morbidity and mortality. Total lymphocyte count, transferring (7days), prealbumin (2 days), and retinol binding protein are more **acute indicators** of nutritional status. **Answer E.**

20) Before surgery, the patient from above appeared very cachectic due to TNF alpha release. All of the following are preoperative signs indicative of poor nutritional status, **except**:

a) A 10 kg weight loss in a 70 kg patient in six months
b) Prealbumin level of 18 mg/dL
c) Albumin level of 2.4 gm/dL
d) Weight less than 85 % of ideal bodyweight

Normal ranges of prealbumin levels are from 16 – 35 mg per dL. Signs of poor nutritional status include acute **weight loss greater than 10 %** in six months, body weight less than 85 % of ideal body weight, and **albumin** level **less than 3.0** gm/dL. **Answer B.**

21) A 65 year old homeless male is admitted through the emergency department after being found unconscious on the street. He is transferred to a general medical floor and given IV fluids. At 3 AM, the medical resident on call is walking by the patient's room and notices him seizing. The resident calls a Rapid Response Team alert and orders several labs and tests including a STAT ECG which shows a polymorphic ventricular tachycardia. Which of the following is the probable cause of his arrhythmia:

a) Hypercalcemia
b) Hypomagnesemia
c) Hypermagnesemia
d) Hypocalcemia
e) Hypokalemia

Normal magnesium levels are 1.5 – 2.5 mg/dL.
Hypomagnesemia can cause symptoms such as weakness, muscle cramps, **neuromuscular excitability**, and **cardiac arrhythmias**. Some common causes are chronic diarrhea, alcoholism, GI fistula, TPN, malabsorption, and drugs such as diuretics. **Answer B.**

22) Regarding fat metabolism, which of the following is correct:

a) Free fatty acid- binding protein binds long-chain fatty acids
b) Medium and short-chain fatty acids enter circulation through lymphatics
c) Long-chain fatty acids enter the circulation through lymphatics along with chylomicrons
d) Unsaturated fatty acids are the preferred fuel source for the liver

Free fatty acid-binding protein binds short and medium-chain fatty acids. **Medium and short-chain** fatty acids enter the circulation through the **portal vein**. Saturated fatty acids (beta-hydroxybutyrate) are the preferred source of energy for the liver. **Answer C.**

23) 23 year old male was a victim of a gunshot wound to his abdomen. Intraoperatively, you identify 20% injury to one segment of his small bowel. Your assistant asks you which layer of the small bowel is the main responsible for holding the stitches:

a) Mucosa
b) Submucosa
c) Muscularis
d) Serosa

The submucosa contains blood vessels, nerves, and lymphatics. It consists of loose filamentous areolar tissue that connects the mucosa and muscularis layers together. The submucosa is the **strongest layer** of the small bowel, and sutures must be through this layer to maintain integrity of any hand sewn anastomosis. **Answer B.**

24) 24 year old male with a history of Crohn's disease is admitted with abdominal pain, diarrhea, and 25 pound weight loss in the last 4 months. He states that he has had multiple small bowel resections, last one being a little over 4 months ago. Which of the following is false regarding short-gut syndrome:

a) Diagnosis of short-gut syndrome is based on length of bowel
b) A low fat diet will help relieve his symptoms
c) Small bowel length of at least 75 cm without an intact ileo-cecal valve will likely prevent this syndrome
d) Small bowel length of at least 50 cm with an intact ileo-cecal valve will likely prevent this syndrome

Diagnosis of short-gut syndrome is **based on symptoms**, not on bowel length alone. A high fat diet will make symptoms worse. The length of the small bowel needs to be at least 75 cm without an intact ileo-cecal valve, and at least 50 cm with an intact ileo-cecal valve. **Answer A.**

25) Regarding respiratory quotient (RQ), which of the following is false:

a) RQ > 1 is indicative of overfeeding
b) RQ is a measurement of energy expenditure, and is calculated as a ratio of O2 consumed over CO2 produced
c) Pure carbohydrate metabolism has a RQ = 1
d) A patient's RQ can be accurately measured using a respirometer

RQ > 1 is indicative of lipogenesis or **overfeeding**, which can lead to CO2 buildup and **difficulty weaning** a patient from the ventilator. **RQ < 0.7** is indicative of ketosis or **starvation**. Pure **fat metabolism** has a **RQ = 0.7**. Pure **protein metabolism** has a **RQ = 0.8**. **Answer B.**

26) The proportion of total caloric intake supplied as fat, during prolonged parenteral nutrition, should be:

a)   20%
b)   40%
c)   60%
d)   80%

Most calories are supplied **as carbohydrate**. Typically, about 4 to 5 mg/kg/day of dextrose is given. Standard solutions contain up to about **25% dextrose**, but the amount and concentration depend on other factors, such as metabolic needs and the proportion of caloric needs that are supplied by lipids. Commercially available lipid emulsions are often added to supply essential fatty acids and triglycerides; **20 to 30% of total calories** are usually supplied **as lipids**. However, withholding lipids and their calories may help obese patients mobilize endogenous fat stores, increasing insulin. **Answer C.**

27) 72 year old male with acute onset redness and pain in his left toe. He asked you what is the precursor of uric acid in patients with gout :

a) Glucose
b) Alanine
c) Purines
d) Glycine

Uric acid is the end product of the metabolism of **purine compounds**. Hyperuricemia can be caused by impaired renal excretion, overproduction of uric acid, and/or by overconsumption of purine-rich foods. **Answer C.**

28) Which of the following stimulates muscle protein synthesis:

a) Insulin
b) Cortisol
c) Catecholamine
d) Glucagon

Hyperglycemia is present **during acute critical illness** due to the catabolic effects of circulating mediators, such as cortisol, catecholamine, and **glucagon**. **Insulin** mediates an **anabolic state** through protein synthesis , hepatic glycogenesis, and lipogenesis. **Answer A.**

29) Regarding protein sparing effect, what is the minimal daily requirement of glucose administration:

a) 25g
b) 50g
c) 75g
d) 100g

Dietary **carbohydrate and fat** provide the **major sources of energy** for support of body protein metabolism. Administration of carbohydrate has a protein-sparing effect in the fasting subject, whereas fat does not, probably mediated in part by increased insulin secretion. Approximately **40 g of proteins** is necessary as a **daily average** intake to maintain Nitrogen balance, and for this purpose, **100 g/day of glucose** is required. **Answer D.**

30) 30 year old male on long term TPN for Crohn's disease presents with anosmia, rash, and decreased taste. The most likely etiology is:

   a) Fatty acid deficiency
   b) Chromium deficiency
   c) Selenium deficiency
   d) Zinc deficiency

   Fatty acid deficiency can also cause cutaneous rash in similar scenario, but **decreased taste sensation** is specific to **zinc**, also known as acrodermatitis enteropathica. **Answer D.**

31) 31 year old cachectic male underwent splenectomy for trauma, was started on enteral feeds on POD1, and advanced rapidly to meet his full nutritional requirement. On POD7 he developed severe respiratory distress. Most likely nutritional deficit responsible for these symptoms is:

   a) Calcium
   b) Magnesium
   c) Phosphate
   d) Potassium

In significantly malnourished patients, the initial stage of oral, enteral, or parenteral nutritional replenishment causes electrolyte and fluid shifts that may precipitate disabling or fatal medical complications. **Hypophosphatemia** is the **hallmark** of the syndrome which can also be associated with **Hypokalemia, Hypomagnesemia, and edema**. **Answer C.**

32) Which of the following is one of the glutamine functions during catabolic stress:

    a) Source of ammonia during urea cycle
    b) Metabolized to glucose by glutaminase
    c) Substrate for immune proliferation
    d) Increased levels in plasma caused by muscle release
    e) Requires enteral delivery to promote intestinal integrity

    It is hypothesized that during stress, glutamine **may preserve immune cell and enterocyte function** and enhance nitrogen balance. **Answer C.**

7. FLUID, ELECTROLYTES AND ACID-BASE BALANCE

1) Which of the following compartments contains the largest percentage of total body water (TBW):

   a) Extracellular
   b) Intracellular
   c) Vascular
   d) Plasma

   TBW is about **60%** of body weight. The intracellular compartment contains 2/3 of total body water. The extracellular compartment contains 1/3 and is split into intravascular and extracellular with ¼ being intravascular and ¾ being extracellular fluid. **Answer B.**

2) What is the electrolyte composition of Lactated Ringer's solution:

   a) Na 154 Cl 154
   b) Na 130 Cl 109 K 4 Ca 3 lactate 28
   c) Na 145 Cl 145
   d) Na 154 Cl 109 K 8 lactate 35

   A is normal saline, B is Lactated Ringer's, and C is albumin. **Answer B**.

3) A patient has a Na of 150, glucose of 180, and BUN of 11.2. What is his plasma osmolarity:

   a) 294
   b) 304
   c) 314
   d) 324

   Plasma osmolarity is calculated using the equation (Na x 2) + (Glucose/18) + (BUN/2.8). **Answer C.**

4) Your patient has a Serum Na of 130, urine Na of 50, Serum Creatinine of 1 and Urine creatinine of 2. What is his approximate FeNa:

a) 10
b) 15
c) 20
d) 25

FeNa is calculated using the equation Urine Na/Creatinine divided by Plasma Na/Creatinine. **Answer C.**

5) What is the FeNa in a person with prerenal azotemia:

a) <1%
b) >1%
c) < 2%
d) <0.1%

FENa is typically less than 1% in prerenal disease (indicative of the sodium retention) and above 2% in ATN. The urine Na concentration tends to be low in prerenal disease (<20 meq/L), and high in ATN (>40 meq/L) due, in part, to the tubular injury. **Answer A.**

6) What is the correction for low albumin with respect to calcium:

a) For each gram drop in albumin, the calcium drops 2
b) For each gram drop in albumin, the calcium drops 1.6
c) For each gram drop in albumin, the calcium drops 8
d) For each gram drop in albumin, the calcium drops 0.8

Since 1/2 of the calcium is bound to albumin, when the albumin level is low, the serum calcium level is also low. Total serum calcium decreases by about 0.8 mg for every 1 gram decrease in albumin. **Ionized (free) calcium is unaffected** by changes in albumin. **Answer D.**

7) SICU nurse paged you and mentioned that your diabetic patient is hyperglycemic (1000 mg/dl) and hyponatremic (130 mEq/L). What is this patient corrected Na level:

a) 130
b) 144
c) 154
d) 160

To correct for hyperglycemia, add **1.6 for every 100** glucose above 100. In this patient taking 100 as normal, he is 900 above normal. 9 x 1.6 is 14.4. 130 plus 14.4 is 144.
Answer B.

8) What is the maintenance fluid for the a 40 year old female who is 5'5" and weighs 100 kilograms:

a) 100
b) 110
c) 120
d) 140

100 kg is not this patient's ideal body weight (IBW). Maintenance fluid is based on **IBW**. Calculate IBW for women as 100 lbs for 5 feet and an additional 5 lbs per inch above 5 feet. For men it is 106 lbs for 5 feet and an additional 6 lbs for each inch over 5 feet. This patient therefore should weigh approximately 60 kgs [100 + (5x5)]/2. Then use **4,2,1 rule**. This rule states that for the first 10 kg of body weight, 4 mL of fluid are administered per kg, per hour. For the second 10 kg, 2mL/kg/hr are administered, and for each additional kg over 20 kg, 1 mL/kg/hr should be given. **Answer A.**

9) Which of the following is **not** present in 1L of Ringer Lactate:

a) 5 mEq of potassium
b) 130 mmol/L of sodium
c) 3 mEq of calcium
d) 28 mEq of lactate

Fluid	Na	Cl	K	Ca	Lactate	Dextrose
LR	130	109	4	3	28	0
NS	154	154	0	0	0	0
D5½ NS	77	77	0	0	0	50g

Answer A.

10) A 20 year old marathon runner has just completed a 5 K run and comes to the hospital with severe dehydration. Regarding fluid loss and related fluid replacement, which of the following is false:

a) Sweat loss should be replaced with normal saline solution
b) Colitis with severe diarrhea should be replaced with lactated ringer's solution
c) Profuse nausea and vomiting should be replaced with lactated ringer's solution
d) High output small bowel fistula should be replaced with lactated ringer's lactate.

Fluid loss related to profuse nausea and vomiting and sweat loss should be replaced with normal saline. Maintenance IV fluid for gastric losses is replaced with D5 ½ normal saline with 20 mEq of potassium. Bolus of normal saline with potassium included should be avoided as this can result in cardiac arrest. Most **GI losses distal to the pylorus** should be replaced with **lactated ringer's** solution. **Answer C.**

11) A surgical intern is performing AM rounds on a 69 year old male 48 hours after a hemicolectomy for colonic adenocarcinoma. What is the correct fluid replacement for this patient at this time:

a) Lactated ringers
b) Normal saline with 20 mEq K+
c) ½ Normal saline with 20 mEq K+
d) D5 ½ normal saline with 20 mEq K+

During an operation and up to the first 24 hours after trauma/stress (also known as **"resuscitation phase"**), **lactated ringers** should be the fluid of choice. After this period, **maintenance fluid** should be started, ideally **D5 ½ normal saline with 20 mEq K+**. The sugar in the fluid will stimulate insulin release and therefore amino acid uptake and protein synthesis (anabolism). **Answer D.**

12) A 21 year old male with worsening pulmonary function, had rapid sequence intubation 48 hs after suffering a burn injury to approximately 25% of his upper body. Subsequently, while in the ICU, the patient goes into cardiac arrest. What is the most likely cause of his arrest:

a) Acute hyponatremia from fluid replacement therapy
b) Drug overdose
c) Hyperkalemia
d) Massive pulmonary embolism

Hyperkalemia following **succinylcholine** administration can be seen with **burn patients** and **spinal cord injuries**. The upregulation of nicotinic acetylcholine receptors in skeletal muscle is the etiology behind this electrolyte imbalance. With the receptor upregulation, more ion channels are available to release potassium during depolarization. For acute injuries (less then 24hs), many authors would not contraindicate succinylcholine use. **Answer C.**

13) In the patient above, all of the following are true about the treatment for hyperkalemia, **except**:

a) Administer 1 amp of 50% dextrose and 10 units of insulin first
b) Administer 1 amp of calcium gluconate
c) Administer 15 gm of kayexalate
d) Dialysis can be used for refractory hyperkalemia

Calcium gluconate should be administered first to **stabilize the cardiac membrane**. 1 amp of **50% dextrose** and 10 units of **insulin** should be given after the calcium gluconate to drive **K+ into cells** with glucose. Kayexalate exchanges Na+ for K+ and is excreted in feces. **Answer A.**

14) A 65 year old female currently receiving chemotherapy for poorly differentiated lymphoma, presents to the emergency room via EMS having suffered a seizure while at home. The patient has never experienced a seizure in the past and lab work is ordered. Tumor lysis syndrome results in all of the following, **except**:

a) Hyperkalemia
b) Hypercalcemia
c) Hyperuricemia
d) Hyperphosphatemia

Tumor lysis syndrome results in the rapid release of intracellular contents that overwhelm the kidney's excretory capacity. The release of these intracellular contents causes **hyperkalemia, hypocalcemia, hyperuricemia**, and **hyperphosphatemia**. Calcium forms the precipitate calcium phosphate due to the hyperphosphatemia thus resulting in hypocalcemia **Answer B.**

15) A 79 year old male presents to the emergency room from a nursing home with altered mental status. On examination, the 60 kg patient is restless and has dry sticky mucous membranes. A basic metabolic panel is performed that demonstrates a sodium level of 160. Which of the following is his total free water deficit:

a) 7 L
b) 6 L
c) 5 L
d) 4 L

Total free water deficit = 0.6 x patient's weight (kg) x [(Na/140) – 1]
0.6 x 60 x [160/140 – 1] = 5 L
Answer C.

16) A 61 year old female with an 80 pack year smoking history is brought to the emergency department complaining of nausea, vomiting, headaches, and altered mental status. The 50 kg patient is thought to have SIADH from a recently diagnosed small-cell lung cancer. Her current sodium level is 120. Which of the following is the patient's sodium deficit:

a)   300 mEq
b)   400 mEq
c)   500 mEq
d)   600 mEq

Sodium deficit = 0.6 x (weight in kg) x (140 – Na)
0.6 x 50 x (140-120) = 600 mEq
Answer D.

17) An elderly patient is intubated in the ICU for aspiration pneumonia and small bowel obstruction. The ventilated patient has the following arterial blood gas values: pH 7.53, CO2 57, HCO3 38. What is the probable cause of this patient's condition:

a) Acute renal failure
b) NGT suctioning
c) Increased minute ventilation
d) Decreased tidal volume

The patient's ABG represents metabolic alkalosis most likely caused by aggressive nasogastric suctioning. This is usually a **contraction alkalosis** due to **loss of hydrochloric acid** in stomach contents resulting in hypochloremic, hypokalemic, metabolic alkalosis with paradoxical aciduria. **Answer B.**

18) 60 year old male is POD2 s/p mesenteric bypass, on ventilator support with the following settings : FiO2 40%, Respiratory Rate 9, and Tidal Volume 550 ml. This morning, arterial blood gas revealed: pH of 7.28, pO2 100, and pCO2 of 58. Which of the following options corresponds to this patient acid-base disorder:

a) Respiratory acidosis only
b) Metabolic alkalosis with compensatory respiratory acidosis
c) Metabolic and respiratory acidosis
d) Metabolic acidosis only

The **respiratory compensation** to metabolic acidosis results in an approximately **1.2 mmHg decrease in arterial PCO2 for every 1 meq/L reduction in the serum HCO3**. The compensatory response to acute respiratory acidosis causes the serum HCO3 to increase about 1 meq/L for every 10 mmHg elevation in the PCO2. If metabolic acidosis is the primary disorder, an arterial PCO2 substantially higher than the expected compensatory response defines the mixed disorder of metabolic acidosis and respiratory acidosis, while an arterial PCO2 substantially lower, defines the mixed disorder of metabolic acidosis and respiratory alkalosis. **Answer C.**

19) What is the osmolality of Normal Saline solution?

a) 253 mOsm/L
b) 270 mOsm/L
c) 290 mOsm/L
d) 308 mOsm/L

The osmolality of the various resuscitative fluids are: D5W (253), Ringer's lactate (270), 0.9 % NaCl = "normal saline" (308), 5% albumin (290), Hetastarch (310) and 7.5% NaCl (2400). **Answer D.**

20) What is the expected ratio of intravenous volume infusion to intravascular volume expansion for 0.9% NaCl:

a) 1:1
b) 1:3
c) 3:1
d) 2:1

The ratio of intravascular volume infusion to intravascular volume expansion is 3:1 for Ringer's lactate, 8:1 for D5W , 3:1 for 0.9% NaCl, 1:1 for plasma and 5% albumin, and 1:3 for 7.5% NaCl. **Answer C.**

8. TRAUMA/CRITICAL CARE AND BURNS

1) 25 year old male was brought to the emergency department after MVA. During primary survey evaluation, patient was noted to be oriented, verbalizing appropriately and with normal breath sounds. Which of the following is the best predictor of an intact airway:

   a) Having symmetrical, bilateral breath sounds
   b) Absence of tachypnea or bradypnea
   c) Having a normal voice
   d) Having normal inspiration and no wheezes on exam

The primary survey is organized according to the injuries that pose the most immediate risks to life and is performed in the following order. It consists of the following steps:
- **A**irway assessment and protection, while maintaining c-spine stabilization
- **B**reathing and ventilation assessment (maintain adequate oxygenation)
- **C**irculation assessment (control hemorrhage and maintain adequate end-organ perfusion)
- **D**isability assessment (perform basic neurologic evaluation)
- **E**xposure, with environmental control (undress patient and search everywhere for possible injury, while preventing hypothermia)
   A clear and accurate response verifies the patient's ability to mentate, phonate, and to protect their airway, at least temporarily.
   Answer C.

2) Regarding surgical airway control in the pediatric patient, which of the following is the most common contraindication to perform cricothyroidotomy:

a) Limitation to place a tube size 6mm or greater
b) Risk of subglottic stenosis
c) Proximity to blood vessels
d) Inability to convert to formal tracheostomy

Cricothyrotomy is indicated when an emergency airway is required and orotracheal or nasotracheal intubation is either unsuccessful or contraindicated. The airway of a child is funnel-shaped, with the narrowest part located at the cricoid ring rather than at the vocal cords. This narrowing increases the risk for developing **subglottic stenosis** following cricothyrotomy. **Answer B.**

3) 30 year old male presented to the emergency room complaining of shortness of breath after a stab wound to the right 5th intercostal space, at the midclavicular line. Physical exam showed BP 90/55, distended jugular vein, and decreased one sided breath sounds. Next step in management should be:

a) CT scan to rule out pulmonary embolism
b) Chest x-ray
c) Chest tube placement
d) FAST exam

Suspected tension pneumothorax is treated with immediate **tube thoracostomy or needle decompression** using a large angiocatheter (eg, 14 gauge). Acceptable sites for needle insertion include the 2nd or 3rd intercostal space in the midclavicular line or the 5th intercostal space in the midaxillary line. If needle decompression is performed first, it is followed by tube thoracostomy. **Answer C.**

4) The only physical finding in class I shock is:

   a) Increased capillary venous filling time
   b) Slight decrease in blood pressure
   c) Urine output of 20-30 mL/h
   d) Confusion
   e) Decreased pulse pressure

   See next comment. **Answer A.**

5) A victim of a gunshot wound to the abdomen presents to your emergency department. Initially the patient appears anxious but quickly becomes confused and combative. The patient has a pulse rate of 135 beats/minute, respiratory rate of 32 breaths/minute, and a blood pressure of 80/45 mmHg. What is the approximate blood loss of this patient:

   a) < 750 ml
   b) 750-1500 ml
   c) 1500-2000 ml
   d) > 2000 ml

The classification of hemorrhagic shock is as follows:

Parameter	Class			
	I	II	III	IV
Blood loss (%)	<15%	15-30%	30-40%	>40%
Blood loss (ml)	<750	750–1500	1500–2000	>2000
Pulse rate (bpm)	<100	**>100**	>120	>140
Blood pressure	Normal	Ortho-static	**Hypo-tension**	Severe Hypo-tension
Respiratory rate	14–20	20–30	30–40	>35
UOP (ml/hr)	>30	20–30	5–15	Negligible
CNS symptoms	Normal	Anxious	Confused	**Lethargic**

The above patient is confused, tachycardic to 135 beats/minute, tachypneic to 32 breaths/minute, and hypotensive, and is therefore in stage III hemorrhagic shock. In an average size adult patient this represents a blood loss of between 1500 and 2000 mL of blood, or approximately 30-40% of total blood volume. **Answer C.**

6) You were called to evaluate a 7 year old male s/p blunt abdominal trauma. FAST was positive and the patient was hypotensive and tachycardic. Initial fluid resuscitation should be:

a) Lactated Ringer's solution at 20 mL/kg bolus
b) Normal saline at 20 mL/kg
c) 1 unit packed RBC's
d) 2 L Lactated ringers solution bolus

Initial fluid resuscitation in hemorrhagic shock after trauma **in adults** consists of **2 L of isotonic saline** (LR or NS) given as rapidly as possible through peripheral IVs. Large volumes of NS can lead to a nonanion gap hyperchloremic metabolic acidosis and LR can cause metabolic alkalosis, as lactate metabolism generates bicarbonate. **Children** should be bolused with **LR at 20 mL/kg** and if the patient does not respond to **3 boluses**, blood should be transfused (10 mL/kg). **UOP, MAP** around 65 mmHg and/or a SBP around 90 mmHg are usual end-points for fluid therapy. **Answer A.**

7) Patients who transiently responds to fluid resuscitation should be considered to have:

   a) Active hemorrhage
   b) Increased intracranial pressure
   c) Faulty monitoring system
   d) Allergic reaction to medications given during resuscitative period

In the trauma patient, any episode of **hypotension** (defined as a SBP <90 mmHg) is assumed to be caused by **hemorrhage until proven otherwise**. Active hemorrhage with temporary control should be considered and re-evaluation recommended. **Answer A.**

8) Regarding small burns immediate management, irrigation with cool water is thought to work by:

   a) Decreasing local tissue temperature to hault spreading necrosis
   b) Prevent edema, therefore reducing thromboxane production
   c) Decreasing pain associated with burn
   d) Causing vasoconstriction

77

Cool water is thought to prevent edema and thromboxane production, **decreasing the inflammatory response** to injury. Ice or cold water should never be used due to systemic hypothermia and vasoconstriction. Topical agents include: Silver sulfadiazine: wide range of antimicrobial activity, primarily as prophylaxis against burn wound infections. Known to cause **neutropenia**.

Mafenide acetate is an effective topical antimicrobial and can be used in both treating and preventing wound infections. Causes **pain and metabolic acidosis** from carbonic anhydrase inhibition.

Silver nitrate is another topical agent with broad-spectrum antimicrobial activity. Side effects include **electrolyte extravasation** with resulting hyponatremia. **Answer B.**

9) Which of the following parameters indicates failure of weaning from ventilator support:

a) Minute ventilation < 15 L/min
b) NIF > -25 cm H20
c) TV > 5 ml/Kg
d) Rapid Shallow Index > 100

Discontinuation of mechanical ventilation should be considered if the following criterias are met:

a) Reversal of underlying cause of respiratory failure
b) Adequate oxygenation (P/F ratio >150–200 with PEEP <5–8, FiO_2 <0.4–0.5, and pH <7.25)
c) Hemodynamic stability
d) The capability to initiate a respiratory effort

RSBI < 100 predicts 80% success on extubation. Other parameters include PaO2 > 60, pCO2 < 50. RR <30 and PEEP <8. Tidal volume, NIF, and minute ventilation are not well standardized. **Answer D.**

10) 35 year old male was stabbed multiple times in the neck, between the clavicle and cricoid region. Which of the following interventions should not be performed:

a) CT Angiogram
b) Chest X-Ray
c) Flexible esophagoscopy
d) Bronchoscopy

Rigid EGD should be performed. Zone I (Clavicle to cricoids) and Zone III (angle of mandible to skull base) are usually managed conservatively. Zone II should be explored if platysma is violated. Chest radiographs will confirm or rule out a pneumothorax or hemothorax, and tracheal or esophageal penetration may be identified by combined endoscopy of the trachea and esophagus. CTA, formal angiography, or duplex ultrasound may be used to identify arterial injury. Barium esophagram is also not recommended. **Answer C.**

11) 68 year old male presented to the ER s/p MVA, opening his eyes to verbal stimuli, disoriented and withdrawing from painful stimuli. His GCS is:

a) 9
b) 10
c) 11
d) 12

Severe TBI is defined by a GCS of 8 or less (ICP monitoring if abnormalities on CT scan); Moderate TBI is between 9 to 12 and a score of 13 to 15 is considered a minor TBI. SBP should be maintained above 90 mm Hg to prevent secondary brain injury and hypotonic fluids can contribute to worsening of brain edema (NS preferred). 2 +4+4 = 10. **Answer B.**

12) 21 year old male, s/p MVA and neck laceration presented to the ER hemodinamically stable, with stridor and subcutaneous air. Gastrograffin study did not show any leak. After airway control, the next step in this suspected esophageal injury include:

   a) Observation
   b) Primary closure
   c) Barium study
   d) Antibiotics and simple drainage

   Gastrograffin study can miss 10-20 % of esophageal perforations. This should be followed by a **thin barium** contrast study. If injury is less then 24hs, primary **2-layer closure**, buttressed with tissue (stomach, pleura or intercostals muscle) and drainage is indicated. If greater than 24hs management include simple drainage and possible spit fistula. **Answer C.**

13) 13 year male presented to the ER with LUQ pain after mechanical fall. Abdominal CT demonstrated a Type IV splenic injury with blush. For this hemodinamically stable patient, management includes all of the following, except:

   a) ICU admission for observation
   b) IV fluids and pRBC as needed
   c) Immediate Splenectomy
   d) Angioembolization

   Stable patients who have high-grade splenic injuries on CT scan or signs of **ongoing bleeding** (increasing blood transfusion requirements, blush) may be candidates for **angioembolization**. **Unstable** patients should undergo **splenectomy** or attempts at splenic repair if appropriate. Most splenic injuries can be managed conservatively. **Answer C.**

14) 41 year old male presented to the ER after falling from a ladder. Intra operatively a liver laceration was found with active bleeding. Patient was transfused several units of pRBC's and FFP's but Pringle maneuver failed to control the bleeding. Next step should be:

a) Kocher maneuver
b) Aortic clamp
c) Packing and transfer to the ICU
d) Transfuse factor 7 and angioembolization

Liver bleeding that is not controlled with Pringle maneuver most likely comes from the hepatic veins. This patient most likely is also coagulopathic (hypothermia, acidosis, hypocalcemia from blood transfusion) and should be resuscitated for 24 hs in the ICU before attempting to control the lesion (Damage Control). **Answer C.**

15) 51 year old male had a gunshot wound to his back and CT scan showed pancreatic laceration. Which of the following test best predicts ductal injury:

a) Triple phase CT abdomen/pelvis
b) ERCP
c) MRCP
d) Endoscopic Ultrasound

When injury involves the pancreatic duct (Grade III), surgery is usually indicated. Options include distal pancreatectomy, Roux-en-Y pancreaticojejunostomy and Whipple procedure (rarely performed for combined duodenum injury). Even though MRCP can be performed, the best test to evaluate ductal involvement is an ERCP. **Answer B.**

16) 16 year old male was brought to the Emergency Department s/p gunshot wound to the abdomen. Intra operatively, patient was hemodinamically stable and a right colon perforation was noted. Appropriate management is:

a) Total colectomy with ileo-rectal anastomosis
b) Total colectomy with ileo-rectal anastomosis and protective ileostomy
c) Right hemicolectomy with primary anastomosis
d) Subtotal colectomy

Except for the unstable patient that requires damage control operation, **most colonic injuries** should be **primarily repaired**. Simple laceration should be debrided and closed, and more complex lacerations should be resected and anastomosed primarily. **Answer C.**

17) A 71 year-old man is rescued from an apartment fire and transported to the trauma center. Physical examination demonstrates 2nd degree burns to the anterior surface of his chest and abdomen, as well as his entire right arm and both legs. An estimate of the total burn surface area of this patient is:

a) 30-34%
b) 35-39%
c) 40-44%
d) 45-49%
e) 50-54%

The **rule-of-9's** is a commonly tested method of calculating total burn area. For an adult patient, total burn area is approximated as follows: Each upper extremity → 9%; Anterior or Posterior chest → 9% each; Anterior abdomen or back → 9% each; Anterior or posterior leg → 9%; Head →9%; Genitalia → 1%.

This patient has received burns to (9 + 9 + 9+ 9 + 9) = 45% of his body. **Answer D.**

18) The above patient is found to weigh 80kg. What is the appropriate initial fluid resuscitation:

a) NS 12.6L in 1st 24 hrs, with 6.3L administered in the 1st 8 hrs
b) LR 12.6L in 1st 24 hrs, with 6.3L administered in the 1st 8 hrs
c) NS 14.4L in 1st 24 hrs, with 7.2L administered in the 1st 8 hrs
d) LR 14.4L in 1st 24 hrs, with 7.2L administered in the 1st 8 hrs
e) NS 16.2L in 1st 24 hrs, with 8.1L administered in the 1st 8 hrs

The **Parkland formula**, which is used to estimate initial fluid resuscitation requirements, when total burns are 20% of total surface area or greater. Appropriate fluid resuscitation is **4cc per kg body weight times the estimated burn area**.

Lactated Ringer's is the solution of choice, with half given in the first eight hours and the balance given over the next sixteen hours. **Answer D**.

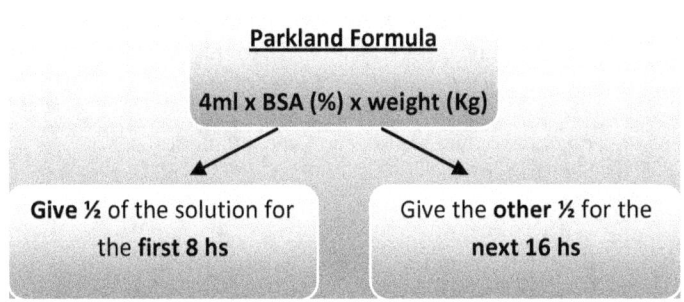

19) Thirty minutes later the paramedics deliver the above patient's granddaughter whom he was babysitting at the time of the fire. The child suffered 2nd degree burns to the anterior chest and abdomen, the entire right leg, as well as the lower half of the left leg. What is the estimated total burn area:

a) 30-34%
b) 35-39%
c) 40-44%
d) 45-49%
e) 50-54%

It's important to remember that the rule-of-9's is different for adults and infants. Because the **heads of infants are disproportionately large** compared to overall body surface area, the rule-of-9's must be modified. For infants and small children the head is approximately **18% of total body area**, twice the value in adults, and the **legs are 14% each**, slightly less than that seen in adults. The remainder of the rule-of-9's remains consistent. This child suffered $(18 + 14 + 7) = 39\%$ of her total body area. **Answer B.**

20) The adult patient above has circumferential burns to both legs. You notice the right lower extremity is severely edematous and has decreased capillary refill and pain sensation. What is the proper course of action:

a) Aggressive fluid resuscitation and antibiotics
b) Escharotomy
c) Fasciotomy
d) Stat arteriogram
e) Prep the patient for emergent extra-anatomical revascularization

Formation of a rigid circumferential **eschar can act as a tourniquet**, particularly when involving the extremities, leading **first to venous compromise followed by arterial insufficiency**. Left untreated this may progress to **compartment syndrome**. Escharotomy is rarely indicated within the 1st eight hours and in general should be not be performed prophylactically. However, when indicated, escharotomy may be quickly at the bedside with the use of electrocautery. **Answer B.**

21) Despite performing the indicated decompressive procedure, his symptoms do not improve. In fact, over the next few hours you noticed that the vascular exam in the right lower extremity is worsening, and now the dorsalis pedis pulse is barely palpable. What is the appropriate course of action:

    a) Aggressive fluid resuscitation and antibiotics
    b) Repeat the escharotomy with deeper penetration and extension of the incisions proximally
    c) Fasciotomy
    d) Stat arteriogram
    e) Prep the patient for emergent extra-anatomical revascularization

Compartment syndrome is a potential consequence of circumferential eschar formation. This is evidenced by the **6 P's**; pain, pallor, paralysis, paresthesia, pulselessness, and poikilothermia. When present, simple escharotomy may be insufficient to relieve the pressure and fasciotomy may be necessary. **Answer C.**

22) As part of the follow-up care of the above two patients you applied topical Silvadene to the burn areas. What is a side-effect of this treatment:

a) Leukopenia
b) Hyopnatremia
c) Localized tissue necrosis
d) Metabolic acidosis
e) Type I hypersensitivity reaction

Silvadene (silver sulfadiazine) is a topical antibiotic cream that is **effective against** a wide spectrum of **gram-negative and gram-positive** organisms. It is **sulfa based** and is therefore contraindicated in patients with a sulfa allergy. It is also ineffective against Pseudomonas species and has **poor penetration** into eschars. Silvadene may also cause **neutropenia** (leucopenia) and **thrombocytopenia.** **Hyponatremia** is a common side effect of **silver nitrate.** **Metabolic acidosis** is a common side effect of **mafenide** sodium (Sulfamylon). **Answer A.**

23) Several hours later the fire investigator is brought to the emergency department with odd-appearing burns to both hands. As it turns out, the previous victim was an amateur petrologist (rock collector) and had a sizable supply of hydrofluoric acid in the apartment. One of the containers apparently ruptured and covered the investigator's hands while she was examining the blaze. What is the appropriate therapy for this injury:

a) Localized ice packs to prevent systemic absorption and dissemination of the chemical
b) Intravenous administration of calcium gluconate
c) Topical calcium gluconate gel to the burn area
d) Application of topical sodium bicarbonate to neutralize the acid

Hydrofluoric acid is a common household and industrial solvent that can result in severe chemical burns. When exposed to biologic tissue, fluoride ions cause precipitation of calcium resulting in **localized and systemic hypocalcemia**. This can lead to QT prolongation, torsade de pointes, or even ventricular fibrillation. Hydrofluoric acid burns should be **treated first with copious irrigation** of the exposed area **followed by topical application of a 2.5% calcium gluconate** gel. For **burns to the hands**, **intra-arterial** (not intra-venous) **calcium** gluconate is also a treatment option. **Answer C**

24) A 24 year-old male patient was a restrained driver in a high-speed motor vehicle accident. Despite best medical and surgical management the patient is found to be brain dead. The topic of organ donation is best initiated by:

a) The attending surgeon at the earliest indication of brain death
b) A non-biased physician not involved in the case
c) The attending physician and one other physician not involved in the case
d) The ethics committee
e) A specially trained personnel and not the attending physician or surgeon

The Advisory Committee on Transplant (ACOT) recommends that: "each transplant center identify and provide to each potential donor an independent and trained patient advocate whose primary obligation would be to help donors understand the process, the procedure and risks and benefits of live organ donation". **Answer E.**

25) A post-CABG patient had been intubated and mechanically ventilated in the ICU for several weeks. The SIMV function has been used exclusively for support and now for weaning to extubate. Weaning parameters include all of the following, **except**:

a) Negative inspiratory force (NIF) > 20
b) FiO2 ≤ 50%
c) PEEP and pressure support of 5
d) Heart rate < 120 beats/min and respiratory rate < 24 breaths/min
e) Normal arterial bloog gas

The following parameters are generally indicative of a patient that will tolerate extubation and independent ventilation:

- Negative inspiratory pressure (NIF) > 20
- FiO2 < 35%
- PEEP of 5 (physiologic)
- Pressure support ≤ 5
- Respiratory rate < 24 breaths/minute
- Heart rate < 120 beats/minute
- Normal arterial blood gases (ABGs)
  - ☐ pH 7.35-7.45
  - ☐ PCO2 < 50 mmHg
  - ☐ PO2 > 60 mmHg
  - ☐ SpO2 ≥ 92%
- Able to follow commands (able to lift and support head off pillow for short periods of time)
  Answer B.

26) A left-shift of the oxygenation dissociation curve is caused by all of the following, **except**:

a) Hypothermia
b) Hypocapnia
c) Decreased 2,3-DPG
d) Acidosis

A right shift of the oxygen dissociation curve results in a decreased affinity of hemoglobin for oxygen, releasing more O2 (**"Right is Right"**). This will require an increased partial pressure of oxygen in the lungs to maintain hemoglobin saturation but will also facilitate greater dissociation of oxygen from hemoglobin in the periphery. A right shift may be caused by the following:

- Increased temperature
- Increased PCO2
- Increased 2,3-DPG
- Increased H+ (Acidosis - decreased pH)

Likewise, a **left shift** results in an **increased affinity** of hemoglobin for oxygen. This results in greater hemoglobin saturation in the lungs at lower O2 partial pressures but also inhibits oxygen unloading in the tissues. A left shift may be caused by the following:

- Decreased temperature
- Decreased PCO2
- Decreased 2,3-DPG
- Alkalosis (increased pH)

Answer D.

27) You performed a complicated open left hemicolectomy with Hartmann's pouch on a 65 year-old male with bowel obstruction. The procedure took four hours and required extensive dissection in the abdomen and pelvis. Post-operatively the patient has made less than 20ml of urine per hour and his creatinine was 2.6 (from 0.9 preoperatively). What is the most likely etiology of his oliguria:

a) Transection of the ureters
b) Intraoperative hypotension
c) Urethral trauma secondary to Foley catheter placement
d) Sepsis

Hypotension is the most common cause of post-operative acute renal failure (ARF). Surgical patients are particularly vulnerable to hypotension leading to ARF. Insensible fluid losses can be as much as 10cc/kg/day. In addition, patients undergoing **open abdominal procedures can lose** anywhere from **0.5 to 1L of fluid per hour**, not including blood losses. If this fluid is not adequately replaced intra- and postoperative, hypotension associated ARF may occur. **Answer B**.

28) In addition to IV fluids and furosemide challenge, you decide to order stat labs. The following results were noted: Na 140, K 4.3, Cl 109, CO2 21, BUN 55, Cr 2.6, Glucose 98, urine Na 14, urine Cr 28. Which of the following is his fractional excretion of sodium (FeNa):

a) 0.85-0.90%
b) 0.91-0.95%
c) 0.96-1.0%
d) 1.01-1.05%
e) 1.06-1.1%

Calculating the FeNa is a useful means of determining whether renal failure is due to prerenal, postrenal, or intrinsic pathology. **Prerenal** acute kidney failure is suggested with a **FeNa of <1%**, whereas intrinsic and postrenal failure demonstrate FeNa values of >1% and >4%, respectively. FeNa is calculated as follows:

$$FeNa = (urine\ Na/Cr)/(plasma\ Na/Cr).$$

In the above case the FeNa is $(14/28)/(140/2.6) = 0.93\%$. This supports a prerenal etiology for this patient's acute renal failure. **Answer B**.

29) A child is brought to the emergency department after having been struck in the abdomen with a baseball bat during a T-ball tournament. Patient was hemodinamically stable and Abdominal CT scan with IV contrast demonstrates blunt spleen trauma with a "blush". What is the most appropriate treatment:

   a) Diagnostic laparoscopy and splenectomy
   b) Emergent exploratory laparotomy and splenectomy
   c) Emergent exploratory laparotomy and splenic salvage
   d) Angiography with coil embolization
   e) Non-operative management

   In any patient, the presence of a **splenic blush** on CT scan following blunt force abdominal trauma is an indication of **active bleeding** and therapeutic options are interventional radiology **embolization** or operative repair. The threshold for splenectomy is the **hemodynamic status**, and most stable patients respond favorably to **conservative management. Answer E.**

30) An unrestrained driver involved in a motor vehicle accident is delivered to your emergency department by the local fire department. The patient withdraws from pain, has no verbal responses whatsoever, and opens his eyes briefly only to painful stimuli. What is this patient's Glasgow Coma Scale (GCS) score:

   a) 6
   b) 7
   c) 8
   d) 9
   e) 10

The Glasgow Coma Scale (GCS) is a means of quantifying a patient's state of consciousness and is useful for directing initial therapy. The scale is calculated as follows:

Motor	
• Follows commands	6 pts
• Localizes pain	5 pts
• Withdraws from pain	4 pts
• Decorticate posturing (flexion with pain)	3 pts
• Decerebrate posturing (extension with pain)	2 pts
• No response	1 pt
Verbal	
• Oriented	5 pts
• Confused	4 pts
• Inappropriate response	3 pts
• Incomprehensible sounds	2 pts
• No response	1 pt
Eye opening	
• Spontaneous opening	4 pts
• Opens eyes on command	3 pts
• Opens eyes to pain stimuli	2 pts
• No eye opening	1 pt

The maximum GCS score is 15 points while the minimum score is 3 points. In general, a GCS score **≤ 14 warrants a head CT, ≤ 10 warrants intubation**, and **≤ 8 warrants intracranial pressure monitoring**.

The patient withdraws from pain (4 pts), has no verbal responses (1 pts), and opens his eyes briefly only to painful stimuli (2 pts), for a total of 7 points. In addition to head CT scan and intubation this patient requires ICP monitoring. **Answer B.**

31) In assessing this patient you place a subdural screw in order to monitor his intracranial pressure (ICP). Which of the following options describes the correct formula to calculate the cerebral perfusion pressure and the normal ICP range:

a) Systolic blood pressure minus intracranial pressure; 5-10mmHg
b) Diastolic blood pressure minus intracranial pressure; 5-10 mmHg
c) Systolic blood pressure minus intracranial pressure; 15-20mmHg
d) Mean arterial pressure minus intracranial pressure; 7-15mmHg
e) Mean arterial pressure minus intracranial pressure; 15-20mmHg

Cerebral perfusion pressure (CPP) is calculated as follows:
CPP = (MAP) − (ICP)
Normal ICP in a supine patient is **7-15 mmHg**. ICPs of 20-25 mmHg or greater require intervention to prevent uncal or tonsillar herniation. CPP is an important parameter in that a low CPP can result in brain ischemia while excessively high CPP can result in increased ICP. Normal CPP is between 60-90 mmHg. **Answer D.**

32) Secondary survey of the above patient demonstrates no blood at the urethral meatus and a Foley catheter was inserted. Immediately afterwards 800ml of grossly bloody urine is drained. Follow-up cystogram demonstrates an extraperitoneal bladder rupture. What is the appropriate management of this injury:

a) Immediate removal of the Foley catheter followed by operative repair of the bladder injury
b) Maintain the Foley catheter in place and prep for operative repair of the bladder injury
c) Suprapubic catheter placement followed by operative repair of the bladder injury
d) Placement of bilateral ureteral stents followed by operative repair of the bladder injury
e) Maintain Foley catheter for 7-10 days and reassess the injury

Bladder injury is indicated by the triad of **gross hematuria**, **suprapubic pain**, and **inability to void**. Once urethral injury is ruled out by retrograde urethrogram, cystogram is the test of choice to assess for bladder injury. Whereas intraperitoneal bladder rupture requires surgical repair, **extraperitoneal injuries** are best managed conservatively with a **Foley catheter for 7-10 days** followed by reassessment. Greater than 85% of extraperitoneal bladder injuries will heal within 3 weeks, though a minority of cases may eventually require surgical repair. **Answer E.**

33) In which of the following receptors does vasopressin binds to cause vasoconstriction:

a) V1
b) V2
c) V3
d) V4

There are multiple receptors for vasopressin ADH. The **V1a and V1b** receptors primarily mediate the **vasoconstriction** response and **ACTH release**, while **V2** receptors principally cause **antidiuretic** effect. **Answer A.**

34) 34 year old male was admitted 4 days ago with 35% total body surface second degree burn, now with cellulitis around the groin burn area. Which of the following is/are required to establish the diagnosis of wound infection in this patient:

a) Qualitative culture
b) Quantitave cultures
c) Wound biopsy
d) Blood cultures
e) A and B
f) B and C

Quantitative wound cultures and **histopathology** are required to establish the diagnosis of a bacterial infection, **>10^5 bacteria** or microbial invasion, respectively. **Colonization** is defined as <10^5 bacteria/gram tissue cultured from the wound surface. The most common pathogens for burn infections and sepsis include MSSA, MRSA, and Pseudomonas aeruginosa. **Answer F.**

35) Which of the following urine findings is expected when the patient develops Hepatorenal syndrome:

a) Potassium lower than 10 mEq/L
b) Potassium greater than 50 mEq/L
c) Sodium greater than 50 mEq/L
d) Sodium lower than 10 mEq/L

HRS is considered a **severe form of prerenal azotemia** that does not respond to volume repletion in the presence of advanced liver failure. Oliguria and a low FE_{Na} are frequent. **Answer C.**

36) Oxygen content is most dependent on:

a) 2.3 DPG level
b) Hemoglobin level
c) PH
d) PaO2

The arterial oxygen content (CaO_2) is the amount of oxygen bound to hemoglobin plus the amount of oxygen dissolved in arterial blood:
CaO_2 (mL O_2/dL) = (1.34 x **Hb** concentration x **SaO$_2$**) + (0.0031 x **PaO$_2$**). **Answer B.**

37) Which of the following risk factors for Acute Respiratory Distress Syndrome is the most prevalent:

a) Sepsis
b) Pulmonary contusion
c) Blood transfusion
d) Gastric aspiration

More than 50 possible causes have been identified and sepsis is the most common cause of ARDS. Consequences include **decreased compliance** , increased pulmonary arterial pressure, and **impaired gas exchange. Answer A.**

38) Which of the following is **NOT** part of the Surviving Sepsis Campaign Guidelines:

a) Mean arterial pressure ≥55 mmHg
b) Urine output ≥0.5 mL/kg/h
c) Mixed venous or Central venous oxygen saturation 65 or 70%, respectively
d) CVP 8-12mmHg

Several randomized studies, initiated within 24 h of sepsis onset, demonstrated that resuscitation targeting specific physiologic endpoints **improved mortality** compared to standard resuscitation. The Surviving Sepsis Campaign Guidelines suggested the above mentioned goals with a MAP ≥ 65mmHg during the first 6 hours of resuscitation **(Early Goal Directed Therapy)**. **Answer A.**

39) Which of the following options has the INCORRECT association between Drug/mechanism of action:

a) Epinephrine: Alpha1, Beta 1 and Beta 2 agonist. Low doses increase cardiac output.
b) Norepinephrine: Alpha1 and Beta1 agonist. Potent vasoconstrictor. Increases MAP.
c) Phenylephrine: Alpha adrenergic only. Increases SVR and MAP.
d) Dobutamine: Beta 1 adrenergic. Increases inotropy, chronotropy and left ventricular filling pressure.
e) Isoproterenol: Beta 1 and Beta 2 agonist. Causes vasodilation and decrease in MAP.

Dobutamine is mainly an inotrope that causes vasodilation. This drug is most commonly used in cardiogenic shock and mechanism of action include inotropy and chronotropy augmentation with **decreased** left ventricular filling pressure. Other options associations are correct. **Answer D.**

9. BREAST, SKIN AND SOFT TISSUES

BREAST

1) What is the mechanism of action of tamoxifen:

   a) Competitive inhibitor of estrogen activity in the breast, agonist to estrogen receptor in uterus
   b) Non-competitive inhibitor of estrogen activity in the breast, agonist to estrogen receptor in uterus
   c) Suicide inhibitor in breast, agonist in uterus
   d) Aromatase inhibitor

   Tamoxifen is a selective antagonist of breast estrogen receptors but is a partial agonist of endometrial receptors. Among women with ER-positive breast CA, tamoxifen reduces the risk of recurrence and death when given as adjuvant therapy for early stage disease and can provide palliation in those with metastatic disease. Side effects include: **increased incidence of uterine or endometrial cancers,** Thromboembolic events, Hepatotoxicity, and bone marrow suppression. **Answer A.**

2) Trastuzumab is used to treat HER-2/neu positive breast cancers. What is its mechanism of action:

   a) Competitive inhibition of HER-2/neu
   b) Non-competitive inhibition of HER-2/neu
   c) Monoclonal antibody that selectively binds to human epidermal growth factor receptor 2 protein (HER-2)
   d) Aromatase inhibitor

Trastuzumab (Herceptin) is a **monoclonal antibody** that selectively binds to human EGF receptor, resulting in its destruction intracellularly. There is clear evidence that its addition to a taxane- and/or anthracycline adjuvant chemotherapy regimen reduces disease relapse and death among women with **HER2-positive** early breast cancer. Main side effect is **cardiotoxicity**. **Answer C.**

3) 45 year old female was found to have a 1cm mass on her left breast. Biopsy confirmed LCIS. Which of the following is not an appropriate management of her condition:

a) Bilateral prophylactic mastectomy
b) Quarterly physical exam and annual mammography
c) Mirror biopsy of contralateral breast
d) Endocrine Therapy

LCIS is usually an incidental finding on biopsy, not considered premalignant, but a **marker of increased risk** (8-10fold) of developing invasive carcinoma in either breast. **Surveillance** is the most commonly recommended treatment strategy for biopsy proven LCIS.
Chemoprevention with tamoxifen shows a 50% decrease in the development of invasive CA. Bilateral prophylactic mastectomy is also an option. **Answer C.**

4) BRCA1 and BRCA 2 are found on which of the following chromosomes:

a) BRCA1 17q21, BRCA 2 13q12
b) BRCA1 13q12, BRCA 2 17q21
c) BRCA1 5q3, BRCA2 7q21
d) BRCA1 13q3, BRCA2 5q3

BRCA genes are **tumor suppressor genes** that increase the risks for breast and ovarian CA (**autosomal dominant**). It is responsible for 5-10% of all cancers and carry a lifetime risk of 40-85% for developing breast CA.

BRCA 1 – As with breast CA, the risk of ovarian CA is higher in women with BRCA1. Carriers also have elevated risks for cervix, uterus, pancreas, gastric, prostate cancers.

BRCA 2 - In men, the lifetime risk of breast CA is ~ 10% and prostate CA is 5-7 fold. Carriers may have elevated risks of gall bladder, bile duct, prostate, pancreas, and gastric CA, as well as melanoma.

Tamoxifen shows a 50% risk reduction in developing cancer and **bilateral mastectomy** decreases risk by 90–94%. **Answer A.**

5) 24 year old female had a breast biopsy performed that showed Cystosarcoma phylloides. Metastatic work up was negative. Appropriate surgical therapy is:

a) Excision with 1cm margin followed by adjuvant therapy
b) Excision with 2cm margin followed by adjuvant therapy
c) Excision and chemoradiation
d) Excision with 1cm margin

Cystosarcoma phylloides/phylloides tumor is **similar to fibroadenoma** except that it has increased cellularity and mitotic rate. **Malignant potential** is determined by mitotic rate. Excision alone with 1cm margin is adequate. Larger tumors may require mastectomy. Half of excised tumors may recur locally, in which case mastectomy is the treatment of choice. **Answer D.**

6) Which of the following lesions predisposes to breast cancer:

a) Sclerosing adenosis
b) Atypical ductal hyperplasia
c) Fibroadenoma
d) Florid hyperplasia

Ductal hyperplasia with atypia is considered a **premalignant lesion**. Sclerosing adenosis is a proliferative disease without atypia and it does not increase cancer risk. Fibroadenoma is a non proliferative breast disease with no malignant potential. **Answer B.**

7) 60 year old female had a left breast stereotactic biopsy last week and Breast cancer was confirmed. What is the most likely pathology report:

   a) Invasive lobular
   b) Invasive ductal
   c) Inflammatory
   d) Ductal carcinoma in situ

   Breast CA is the most common female CA in the US and the 2nd most common cause of CA death in women. **Infiltrating ductal carcinoma is the most common type** of invasive breast CA (70-80%). Most breast cancers arise from the ductal cells. DCIS is a premalignant lesion. **Answer B.**

8) 75 year old female returns to your office 1 week after modified left mastectomy complaining of pain and weakness on the ipsilateral extremity. You suspect serratus palsy. Which of the following nerve was most likely injured:

   a) Thoracodorsal nerve
   b) Axillary nerve
   c) Long thoracic nerve
   d) Medial pectoral nerve

The **Long thoracic nerve** innervates the serratus anterior muscle and patients with **serratus injury** may present with pain, weakness, and **scapular winging**. **Axillary Nerve** innervates the deltoid, teres minor, and triceps brachii long head resulting in **loss of abduction** 15 to 90 degrees and weak flexion. **Thoracodorsal nerve** innervates the **latissimus dorsi** and injury causes inability to do a **pull-up**. Medial pectoral innervates the pectoralis major and minor. **Answer C.**

9) During sentinel lymphnode biopsy, which of the following is a potential complication of lymphazurin blue dye injection:

a) Type I hypersensitivity reaction
b) Type II hypersensitivity reaction
c) Type III hypersensitivity reaction
d) Type IV hypersensitivity reaction

Lymphazurin can result in Type I hypersensitivity reaction in 1% of patients. **Answer A.**

10) Which of the following is **NOT** a contraindication to sentinel lymph node biopsy:

a) Pregnancy
b) Multicentric disease
c) Palpable lymph nodes
d) Tumor greater than 1cm

SLND is indicated for T1, T2 tumors to assess the regional lymph nodes in women who are clinically node negative. Contraindications include T3, T4, or inflammatory breast CA, tumors greater than 5cm, tumors with clinically positive nodes, pregnancy, and DCIS without mastectomy planned. **Answer D.**

11) A 54 year old male with a history of Klinefelter syndrome presents with a left subareolar mass. Regarding male breast cancer, which of the following is false:

a) Conditions that are associated with an increased level of estrogen, such as Klinefelter syndrome and cirrhosis, increases risk of breast cancer in men
b) The most common type of breast cancer in men is infiltrating lobular carcinoma
c) Breast conserving surgery with sentinel lymph node biopsy may be performed if the axilla is clinically negative for lymphadenopathy
d) BRCA 2 mutation is associated with an increased risk of male breast cancer

The **most common** type of breast cancer in men and women is **infiltrating ductal cancer**. Although most men undergo modified radical mastectomy for breast cancer, **men with large breasts** who are clinically negative for axillary lymphadenopathy **may undergo BCT** (lumpectomy with SLN biopsy). **Answer B.**

12) A 34 year old pregnant patient is diagnosed with invasive ductal carcinoma of the left breast. She is in her second trimester of pregnancy. Which of the following option is a false statement:

a) Radiation therapy is contraindicated until after delivery
b) Modified radical mastectomy is indicated during the 1st and 2nd trimester of pregnancy
c) Chemotherapy can be administered during the 1st trimester of pregnancy.
d) Pregnant women have a similar prognosis, stage for stage, in comparison to women who are not pregnant.

Chemotherapy during the **1st trimester** of pregnancy is associated with **spontaneous abortions** and congenital defects, but it can be administered during the 2nd and 3rd trimesters. **Answer C.**

13) Which of the following is false regarding anastrazole, an aromatase inhibitor:

   a) Anastrazole is preferred over tamoxifen for post menopausal women.
   b) A side effect of anastrazole is deep vein thrombosis.
   c) Anastrazole prevents the peripheral conversion of fats to estrogen.
   d) Anastrazole is associated with bone loss.

   Aromatase inhibitors do not have partial agonist activity, in contrast to **tamoxifen**, consequently, those drugs are not associated with **endometrial CA** and **thromboembolic events**. **Answer B.**

14) The monoclonal antibody, traztuzumab is effective in patients with:

   a) ER receptor
   b) PR receptor
   c) HER2/neu receptor
   d) All three receptors

   Traztuzumab **increases the survival rate** in HER2/neu receptor positive patients. This interaction results is **cellular growth inhibition**. **Cardiac toxicity** is the main side effect. **Answer C.**

15) Which of the following statements regarding breast cancer staging is false:

a) T3 lesion is >2 cm and <5cm in greatest dimension
b) N1 refers to metastasis to movable ipsilateral lymph nodes
c) N2 refers to metastasis to fixed ipsilateral lymph nodes
d) Ipsilateral internal mammary lymph node metastasis is classified as N3

TNM	Description
T1	Tumor size $\leq$ 2cm
T2	Tumor size $\geq$ 2cm but $\leq$ 5cm
T3	Tumor size $\geq$ 5cm
T4	Direct invasion to chest wall or skin
N1	Movable ipsilateral lymph nodes
N2	Fixed ipsilateral lymph nodes
N3	Ipsilateral infraclavicular lymph nodes

Answer A.

16) Which of the following option is the treatment option for Mondor's disease of the breast:

a) NSAID's
b) Incision and drainage
c) Mammogram
d) Excisional biopsy

Mondor's disease is a **superficial thrombophlebitis** that presents with a tender cord like structure. Common causes include **infections, trauma**, and surgical interventions. **Warm compresses** and **NSAIDs** are usually all that is necessary. Surgical treatment is rarely indicated. **Answer A.**

SKIN AND SOFT TISSUES

1) Which of the following is the most common skin cancer:

   a) Superficial spreading melanoma
   b) Basal cell carcinoma
   c) Squamous cell carcinoma
   d) Keratoacanthoma

   Nonmelanoma skin cancer is the most common form of
   malignancy in humans. Most common forms on the head
   and neck include basal cell carcinoma,
   squamous cell carcinoma, sebaceous carcinoma, and
   Merkel cell carcinoma.
   BCC- Sun exposure is the most important environmental
   cause. 70% occur on the face. Low metastatic potential, but
   locally invasive. Surgery is the mainstay of therapy (standard
   excision, Mohs micrographic surgery and curettage).
   Answer B.

2) Melanoma comes from what cell type:

   a) Mesenchyme
   b) Neuroectoderm
   c) Stromal cells
   d) Mesoderm

   Melanocytes come from **neuroectoderm** cells. The neural
   crest-derived melanocytes migrate into the epidermis and
   hair follicles during embryogenesis. **Answer B.**

3) Where does melanoma most commonly metastasize:

   a) Small Bowel
   b) Lymph nodes
   c) Brain
   d) Lungs

Most common sites of metastasis, in descending order, are lung, skin, lymph nodes, brain, liver, bone, and GI tract.
Answer D.

4) Which of the following melanoma types is the least aggressive:

a) Nodular
b) Acrallentiginous
c) Superficial spreading
d) Lentigomaligna

The melanomas above are listed in order of aggressiveness from A to D.
Nodular-most aggressive, vertical growth phase melanomas, most likely to have metastasis at diagnosis, bluish black in color.
Acral lentiginous- Least common variant of radial growth phase melanomas. They arise most commonly on palmar, plantar, and subungual regions.
Superficial spreading- most common, sun exposed areas.
Lentigo maligna - Most commonly arises in sun-damaged areas of the skin in older individuals. Radial growth first; least aggressive.

Margins recommended for primary lesion are:

Thickness	Margin
In Situ	0.5-1mm
<1mm	1cm
>1mm	2cm

Wider margins are not associated with increased survival.
Answer D.

5) Main blood supply for transverse rectus abdominal myocutanous (TRAM) flap reconstruction:

a) Superior epigastric vessels
b) Inferior epigastric vessels
c) Internal thoracic vessels
d) Intercostal arteries

The pedicled TRAM flap is based on the **superior epigastric artery and vein**, and is rotated into the breast pocket with the superior portion of the muscle still attached to the costal margin The epigastric vessels are kept intact during a TRAM flap to maintain viability. **Answer A.**

6) How do skin grafts initially receive oxygenation and nutrition:

a) Capillary revascularization
b) Resorption of nutrients and oxygen from extracellular fluid from the surrounding tissue.
c) Active transport
d) Does not require nutrient it is non viable tissue serving as bridge for neoepithelization.

Imbibition is the initial process of oxygenation and nutritional support for a skin graft until revascularization occurs. It is characterized by **resorption of nutrients and oxygen** from extracellular fluid from the surrounding vascularized tissue. **Answer B.**

7) Regarding soft tissue sarcomas, which of the following is the best predictor of local recurrence:

a) Surgical margins
b) Tumor size
c) Histologic grade
d) Positive lymph nodes

The most important **prognostic factor** is the **pathologic stage** at the time of diagnosis. **Staging** is based on the **TNM** system. Although **histologic grade** and **tumor size** are the most important, other factors influence prognosis, including anatomic site, patient age, and histologic subtype. Core needle biopsy is considered the preferred method to achieve an initial biopsy in most cases. **Answer A**.

8) A 61-year-old female undergoes a core needle biopsy of a 1.5 cm mass in her right thigh. All of the following are true, **except**:

a) Most lower extremity sarcomas $\geq$ 1cm require an amputation
b) Only 2-3% of sarcomas metastasize to the lymph nodes
c) Sarcomas are susceptible to radiation and chemotherapy
d) Simple enucleation has a higher rate of recurrence compared to excision with negative margins

Soft tissue sarcomas usually present as an enlarging, **painless mass** in the extremities or trunk. **Diagnosis** is based on **MRI** and **core needle biopsy** (incisional biodsy may be required). **Lung metastases** are the most common (**hematogenous spread**). **Limb sparing** surgeries are the standard of care for extremity sarcomas. However, amputations are acceptable for tumors with invasion to the bones, nerves, and/or vessels. **Answer A.**

9) Which of the following statements is false regarding sarcomas:

a) Thorotrast is associated with increased risk for hepatic angiosarcoma.
b) Chronic lymphedema is associated with increased risk for lymphangiosarcoma.
c) Radiation is associated with increased risk for osteosarcoma.
d) Most sarcomas are associated with an environmental carcinogen.

Most sarcomas **do not have a clearly defined etiology**. They are thought to **arise de novo**, not from a preexisting lesion. 80% originate from soft tissue and the rest from the bones. **Answer D.**

10) What is the most common histologic type of soft tissue sarcoma in adults:

a) Malignant fibrous histiocytoma
b)Leiomyosarcoma
c) Liposarcoma
d)Rhabdomyosarcoma

Malignant fibrous histiocytoma is the most common sarcoma in adults. Rhabdomyosarcoma is the most common soft tissue sarcoma of childhood. **Answer A.**

10. SURGICAL ENDOCRINOLOGY

PITUITARY/ADRENAL GLAND

1) 32 year old female presents to the ER complaining of diplopia and milky drainage from both breasts. Appropriate options include all of the following, except:

a) Beta-HCG and observation
b) Transnasal resection
c) Craniotomy
d) Cabergoline

Prolactinomas are the most common pituitary tumors. Hyperprolactinemia presents with **galactorrhea, infertility, hypogonadism, and amenorrhea**. Diagnosis is usually based on H&P, MRI, and hormone testing.
Treatment depends on their size, hormonal levels, and invasiveness. Micro or macroadenomas that are nonsecreting and are not causing symptoms of compression may be treated conservatively and followed with serial imaging. Cabergoline is a selective D-2 dopamine **receptor agonist. Answer B**.

2) After bilateral adrenalectomy patient has visual problems and amenorrhea. Most likely diagnosis is:

a) Nelson's syndrome
b) Waterhouse-Friderichsen syndrome
c) Sheehan syndrome
d) Craniopharyngioma

Waterhouse-Friderichsen syndrome is **adrenal hemorrhage** that typically occurs after **meningococcal sepsis** and can lead to adrenal insufficiency. **Sheehan** syndrome typically occurs **after pregnancy** that is complicated by hemorrhage. First sign is usually **difficulty lactating. Answer A**.

3) Which of the following options describes the diseases characteristics of MEN I:

a) Pituitary adenoma, pheochromocytoma, parathyroid hyperplasia
b) Pituitary adenoma, medullary carcinoma, parathyroid hyperplasia
c) Pituitary adenoma, parathyroid hyperplasia, pancreatic islet cell tumor
d) Pancreatic adenoma, parathyroid hyperplasia, mucosal neuromas

MEN I consist of pituitary tumors, parathyroid hyperplasia, and pancreatic islet cell tumors. MEN IIa consists of parathyroid hyperplasia, pheochromocytoma, and medullary carcinoma. MEN IIb consists of pheochromocytoma, medullary carcinoma, and mucosal neuromas. **Answer C.**

4) Treatment strategy for prolactinoma includes:

a) Bromocriptine
b) 5-FU
c) Growth hormone
d) Surgery

Bromocriptine is a **dopamine agonist** that inhibits secretion of prolactin. Treatment consists of conservative therapy for nonsecreting microadenomas and macroadenomas without **symptoms of compression**, medical therapy for prolactinomas, and transsphenoidal surgery for symptomatic disease. Craniotomy and radiation therapy may also be used. **Answer A.**

5) 65 year old male was found to have a non secreting Pituitary macroadenoma during trauma work up after a mechanical fall. Patient denies any symptoms at this time. Appropriate management is:

a) Neurosurgery consult for same admission craniotomy
b) Transsphenoidal resection of the tumor to avoid compression symptoms
c) Conservative management with serial imaging studies
d) Urgent transnasal ablation and hormonal replacement

Micro and Macroadenomas of the Pituitary gland that are **asymptomatic and non secreting** should be treated **conservatively** with follow up CT/MRI studies. **Answer C.**

6) Which of the following is not a cause of primary Adrenal Insufficiency:

a) HIV
b) Amyloidosis
c) Cytomegalovirus
d) Glucocorticoid therapy

Most common cause is autoimmune atrophy and less common causes include Viral and Fungal infections, hemorrhage and metastatic cancer. **Steroid use** is the most common cause of **secondary** adrenal insufficiency. **Answer D**.

7) In regards to adrenal blood supply, which of the following is false:

a) Inferior phrenic artery is one of the two primary arteries that supply the Adrenal glands
b) Right adrenal vein drains into the Inferior Vena Cava
c) Venous drainage is more constant then the arterial supply
d) Left adrenal vein drains into the Left renal vein

Adrenal glands are supplied by the **inferior phrenic** artery, direct branches off the **Aorta** and branches from the **renal artery**. **Answer A.**

8) 35 year old male presented to the ER with history of HTN and mild abdominal pain. CT showed a 6 cm right adrenal mass with low attenuation. Which of the following is true:

    a) Most adrenal incidentalomas are functioning adenomas
    b) If this mass is non functioning , it should be resected
    c) Aldosteronoma may present with hypertension and hyperkalemia
    d) Final needle aspiration is useful in differentiating benign from malignant adrenal tumor

    Most incidentalomas are non functioning. **Aldosteronoma** presents with **HTN, hypokalemia and hormone** excess. Surgical indications include functional adrenal tumor and masses > 5cm. **Answer C.**

9) What is the appropriate sequence of preoperative management for a patient with Pheochromocytoma:

    a) Hydration, Propranolol for 2 weeks, followed by phenoxybenzamine if needed
    b) Propranolol , followed by 2 weeks of phenoxybenzamine and hydration
    c) Doxazosin for 2 weeks , diuretics , followed by propranolol if needed
    d) Doxazosin for 2 weeks, hydration and propranolol if needed

    Alpha blockade should be initiated 2 weeks prior to the procedure, until the patient develops **mild orthostatic hypotension**. Diuretics should be avoided, and if tachycardia persists, B-blockade should be added. Intraoperative hypotension is first managed with fluid replacement therapy. **Answer D.**

10) Which of the following is the most common manifestation of MEN II:

a) Parathyroid Hyperplasia
b) Medullary Thyroid Carcinoma
c) Pheochromocytoma
d) Gastrinoma

MEN IIA – Genetic (RET) predisposition to **MTC** (90%), **pheochromocytoma** (40%), and **parathyroid hyperplasia** (10%). Cutaneous lichen amyloidosis is also part of this syndrome.
MEN IIB - Patients with this condition also tend to have **mucosal neuromas, Marfanoid habitus**, and myelinated corneal nerves. MTC is the most common component and more aggressive than in MEN IIA. **Answer B**.

11) Regarding the surgical anatomy of the adrenal veins, which of the following is false:

a) Left adrenal vein drains into the left renal vein
b) Left adrenal vein drains from the lower pole of the gland
c) Left adrenal vein has shorter length
d) Right adrenal vein drains into the IVC

The **right adrenal vein** is shorter in length, larger in diameter, and it drains **directly into** the posterior aspect of the **IVC**. Venous drainage should be controlled first, and for the above reasons, a **right adrenalectomy is more challenging. Answer C.**

12) In which of the following zones estrogen is produced:

a) Medulla
b) Zona reticularis
c) Zona fasciculata
d) Zona glomerulosa

The adrenal gland is divided into adrenal **cortex** (from **mesoderm**) and adrenal **medulla** (**ectoderm**), and each zone produces specific hormones.

Region	Adrenal gland	Hormones
Cortex	Glomerulosa	Aldosterone
Cortex	Fasciculata	Cortisol
Cortex	Reticularis	Sex hormone
Medulla	Medulla	Catecholamines

Answer B.

13) Eighty-percent of the pituitary gland consists of adenohypophysis. Which of the following pars form the adenohypophysis:

a) Pars distalis
b) Pars tuberalis
c) Remnant of pars intermedia
d) All of the above

The pituiary gland comprises mainly the adenohypophysis(anterior lobe) and the neurohypophysis (posterior). The **adenohypophysis** regulates several physiological processes including stress, growth, and lactation. It receives hypothalamic releasing hormones via portal system and release **ACTH, TSH, FSH, and prolactin**. The **neurohypophysis** is part of the endocrine system and consists mainly of neuronal projections from the hypothalamus, releasing the hormones oxytocin **and** vasopressin. **Answer D.**

14) 35-year old female presents to her PCP with complaints of headaches, blurry vision, and white-colored discharge from her breasts. The best radiologic test to confirm your diagnosis is:

   a) MRI
   b) CT scan
   c) Plain radiograph
   d) PET scan

   For patients with prolactinoma, MRI has now become the first choice for imaging of the pituitary gland. MRI with the IV infusion of gadolinium is able to delineate intrasellar tumors 5mm and above. It can also show the growth extension of larger tumors. Ct scans are able to reveal calcification better than a MRI. **Answer A.**

15) Which of the following CT scan finding is not suggestive of adrenocortical carcinoma:

   a) Size greater than 4 cm
   b) >10 HFU on CT scan
   c) Rapid washout on enhanced CT scan
   d) Irregular borders on CT scan
   e) Necrotic center

Features that are suggestive of adrenocortical carcinoma include size **greater than 4 cm** (which also contributes to central necrosis), **irregular borders**, **highly vascular** (making it hyperintense on T2 weighted MRI and have slow washout on enhanced CT), **rapid growth**, and **greater than 10 HFU** on unenhanced CT scan. **Answer C.**

16) In the pre op holding area, your patient who is scheduled for removal of her pheochromocytoma is evaluated and is found to have a blood pressure of 210/120 mmHg. She has been on phenoxybenzamine for 2 weeks. Which of the following would be an appropriate next step in the management of this patient:

a) Cancel the surgery and send the patient home
b) Proceed with surgery after the patient's blood pressure has been stabilized in the pre op area
c) Add metyrosine and stabilize the patient's blood pressure
d) Convert from planned open procedure to laparoscopic adrenalectomy
e) Proceed with surgery but resuscitate aggressively preoperatively

This patient has malignant hypertension and should not undergo surgery. Adding **metyrosine or a beta blocker** to her regimen with a delay in surgery are safe options. Metyrosine is a tyrosine hydroxylase inhibitor which inhibits the synthesis of catecholamines via the pathway below:

Tyrosine → DOPA→ Dopamine→ Norepinephrine→ Epinephrine

Tyrosine Hydroxylase

Laparoscopic approach can be used for adrenal tumors up to 10 cm in size but conversion to open does not decrease the risk of stroke, bleeding, and myocardial infarction associated with malignant hypertension. Simply cancelling the surgery and sending the patient home is also unsafe.
Answer C.

17) A 25 year old female nurse comes to see you in her office after having a spell where she became hypoglycemic, sweaty and passed out. Your staff is suspicious of Munchausen syndrome despite your patient vehemently denying taking exogenous insulin. Which of the following findings would support your patient's argument:

a) Insulin/Glucose ratio of 0.3
b) Urinalysis that is positive for sulfonylureas
c) Normal C-peptide levels
d) Normal proinsulin levels
e) Insulin/c-peptide ratio >1

Insulinoma is a pancreatic tumor that secretes insulin. Insulin is normally cleared by the liver at a higher rate than c-peptide is cleared by the kidneys. For this reason, the **insulin/C-peptide ratio in normal subjects** should be **less than 1** but will be elevated in surreptitious use of insulin. **Elevated levels** of C-peptide (greater than 2.5 ng/mL) is supportive of **insulinoma**. Patients taking sulfonylureas may exhibit hypoglycemia as well, and these will appear in urinalysis. The insulin/glucose ratio in healthy subjects is usually <0.25. **Answer A**.

18) Which of the following findings is suggestive of Conn's syndrome:

a) Plasma aldosterone to plasma rennin ratio of 10
b) 24 hour urinary aldosterone of 10 mcg/day
c) Hypokalemic metabolic alkalosis
d) Blood pressure not responsive to spironolactone
e) Normal sodium level

Conn's syndrome or **primary aldosteronism** is caused by over secretion of aldosterone. This causes an **elevation in sodium and hypokalemic metabolic alkalosis**. Hypokalemia is not present in all patients with Conn's syndrome, however. Another feature of Conn's syndrome is plasma aldosterone to plasma renin ratio greater than 30. Renin is secreted by the juxtaglomerular cells of the kidney which cleaves angiotensinogen to angiotensin I. AT I is then cleaved to AT II in the lungs by ACE. This causes vasoconstriction. In the normal individual, renin is low in the presence of aldosterone. A 24 hour urine aldosterone level greater than 14 is highly suggestive of Conn's syndrome. **Answer C**.

19) 55 year old male with elevated urine VMA and plasma metanephrines underwent a localization study which revealed normal bilateral adrenal glands. Most likely, this tumor will be found at:

a) Adrenal hilum
b) Aortic bifurcation
c) Bladder
d) Posterior mediastinum

Pheochromocytomas are 10 % bilateral, 98% intra-abdominal, and 90% intra-adrenal. Extra-adrenal tumors are usually within the abdomen and located along the sympathetic chain, the periaortic areas, and at the bifurcation of the aorta. Extra abdominal tumors are found in the posterior mediastinum and it also may arise in the bladder. **Answer B.**

THYROID / PARATHYROID

1) 55 year old male presents with a 2cm palpable left thyroid lobe mass. Hormone levels are normal and USG showed a solid lesion. Next step in management should be:

   a) Total thyroidectomy
   b) FNA
   c) Excisional biopsy
   d) Lobectomy

   FNA is the next diagnostic step for most neck masses. If **not palpable**, USG or CT **guided biopsies** should be performed. It provides only sample for **cytologic analysis**, and no material for evaluation of tissue architecture. Ultrasound is adjunctive and is used to differentiate cystic versus solid lesions. **Answer B**.

2) A 32 year old female presents to your clinic complaining only of a palpable mass in her neck. What is the best initial step:

   a) Excisional biopsy
   b) Incisional biopsy
   c) CT scan
   d) FNA
   e) Ultrasound

   Initially, when presented with an asymptomatic thyroid mass the best test is **ultrasound** to identify **solid versus cystic** masses. If cystic, these can be drained. The fluid need not be sent for pathology unless it is bloody. If the cyst regresses no further treatment is needed. If the cyst recurs then excision is a good option. If the mass is **solid**, thyroid function tests should be ordered and an **FNA** performed. **Answer E**.

3) What is the embryologic origin of the thyroid gland:

a) Rathke's pouch
b) Outgrowth of the 4th pharyngeal arch
c) Floor of the pharynx, foramen cecum
d) 1st pharyngeal pouch

The thyroid is derived from the **foramen cecum**. Rathke's pouch is a depression in the developing roof of the mouth which eventually becomes the anterior pituitary. The 4th pharyngeal pouch gives rise to the parafollicular C cells. The 1st pharyngeal pouch gives rise to the endoderm of the auditory canal. **Answer C.**

4) What is the blood supply to the parathyroid glands:

a) Inferior thyroid artery
b) Superior thyroid artery
c) Thyroid ima artery
d) Middle thyroid artery

The **inferior thyroid artery** supply blood to **all 4** parathyroid glands and arises from the **thyrocervical trunk**. The superior thyroid artery is the 1st anterior branch of the external carotid. The thyroid ima is present in a small portion of the population and arises from the brachiocephalic trunk. **Answer A.**

5) The superior parathyroid gland is located:

a) Anterior and Lateral to the recurrent laryngeal nerve
b) Posterior and Medial to the recurrent laryngeal nerve
c) Anterior and Medial to the recurrent laryngeal nerve
d) Through the recurrent laryngeal nerve
e) Posterior and Lateral to the recurrent laryngeal nerve

The superior gland is posterolateral to the recurrent laryngeal nerve and the inferior gland is anteromedial to the recurrent laryngeal nerve. Remember AMPL (inferior is AnteroMedial and Superior is PosteroLateral). **Answer E**.

6) Which of the following is **not** true regarding parathyroid hormone:

   a) Increases reabsorption of calcium
   b) Decreases reabsorption of phosphate
   c) Decreased bone resorption
   d) Increased hydroxylation of vitamin D
   e) Is released from the parathyroid glands

PTH increases reabsorption of calcium and decreases reabsorption of phosphate. It also increases colonic absorption of calcium by increased hydroxylation of Vit D. PTH acts indirectly on osteoclasts to increase bone resportion. **Answer C**.

7) What is the most serious complication of thionamide therapy:

   a) Arrhythmia
   b) Anaphylaxis
   c) Agranulocytosis
   d) Diarrhea

PTU and methimazole (thionamides) can cause agranulocytosis in 0.5% of users. PTU inhibits **T4→ T3 conversion** in extrathyroidal tissue. Both can cause N/V, rash, urticaria, arthritis, and fever. **Answer C**.

8) Medullary thyroid carcinoma occurs due to a mutation in which of the following genes:

a) RET
b) p53
c) RB
d) APC

MTC occurs sporadically 75% of the time and in association with MEN 2 the remaining. RET mutations are frequently found in association with the cancer. Medullary CA arises from **parafollicular cells** and therefore measurement of **calcitonin** is useful as a marker and for surveillance. Treatment is **total thyroidectomy**. When sporadic, it is usually one nodule, when associated with **MEN 2** it is usually **bilateral**. Unlike other thyroid cancers, radioactive iodine is useless. **Answer A**.

9) A 40 year old female has a palpable 2 cm mass in the right thyroid lobe. FNA shows psammoma bodies. What is the treatment of choice:

a) Lobectomy
b) Total thyroidectomy
c) Radioactive iodine and external beam radiation
d) Yearly surveillance

Papillary thyroid carcinoma is associated with previous radiation. Lesions less than 1cm are treated with lobectomy and isthmusectomy. **2cm and greater** are treated with **total thyroidectomy**. It **spreads** mainly **via lymphatics** and the presence of palpable nodes mandates modified radical neck dissection with total thyroidectomy. Treatment with **radioactive iodine** will destroy any remaining tissue. Monitor **thyroglobulin levels for recurrence. Answer B.**

10) What is the embryologic origin of the superior parathyroid glands:

a) 2nd pharyngeal pouch
b) 3rd pharyngeal pouch
c) 4th pharyngeal pouch
d) 5th pharyngeal pouch

The **superior** parathyroids arise from the **4th** pharyngeal pouch while the **inferior** parathyroids arise from the **3rd** pharyngeal pouch. **Answer C.**

11) 65 year old male with severe hypercalcemia was diagnosed with primary hyperparathyroidism. Imaging studies confirmed a right inferior parathyroid adenoma. Intraoperatively you are not able to find the inferior gland. Most commonly, the aberrant location is in the:

a) Carotid sheath
b) Thymus
c) Vertebral body
d) Thyroid gland

Missing **superior gland** is usually located at the middle and posterior neck compartments, particularly the **tracheoesophageal groove**. Missing **inferior gland** or supernumerary gland is usually located at the ipsilateral thymus and upper cervical region. Carotid sheath exploration is the next step. **Answer B**.

12) 60 year old female was found to have elevated calcium levels on routine exam. You suspect Primary Hyperparathyroidism. Regarding this condition, which of the following is true:

a) It is usually caused by multiple adenomas
b) It is usually caused by parathyroid carcinoma
c) It is usually caused by a single adenoma
d) It is most frequently a result of MEN syndrome

Primary hyperparathyroidism is usually a **single adenoma** that is discovered on routine chemistry revealing hypercalcemia. Patients are usually asymptomatic. **Treatment** is reserved for the following scenarios: **symptomatic, 1 mg/dl above upper limit** normal serum calcium, 24 hr **urinary calcium greater than 400** mg, **30% reduction in creatinine clearance,** bone mineral density t-score below -2.5, younger than 50 years old. Sestamibi scan and USG are adjunctive modalities for identifying the adenoma. **Answer C.**

13) A patient presents with the following laboratory exam. Calcium 8.9, PTH 75 pg/ml (normal 10-55), and phosphorous 6.3. What is the most likely etiology:

a) Primary hyperparathyroidism from a solitary adenoma
b) Secondary hyperparathyroidism from renal failure
c) Tertiary hyperparathyroidism
d) Multiple myeloma

Primary hyperparathyroidism has **elevated calcium and PTH**. In **secondary** hyperparathyroidism, **PTH is elevated and phosphorus** is usually **elevated** as a result of renal failure. The **calcium may be normal** or slightly elevated. **Tertiary** hyperparathyroidism occurs after long standing secondary hyperparathyroidism and is the result of **hypertrophied parathyroid** glands from long standing stimulation by PTH. The history must tell you about transplant or long standing secondary hyperparathyroidism. **Answer B**.

14) Regarding thyroid function tests, all of the following is true, **except**:

a) TSH is the best test of thyroid function
b) T3 is three times more active than T4
c) Half-life of T4 is 1-3 days
d) Thyroglobulin stores T3 and T4 in colloid

Half life of T3 is 1-3 days and T4 is 7 days. Most **T3 is produced by conversion from T4** in the periphery. **TSH levels is the most sensitive** test of thyroid function. **Answer C**.

15) 35-year-old female presents to your office complaining of tremors, weight loss and palpitations. Physical exam confirmed an enlarged thyroid gland. Regarding this condition, all of the following is true, **except**:

a) Diffuse goiter with high radiolabel uptake is usually found
b) Grave's disease is the most common cause
c) Caused by autoimmune IgM antibody to the TSH receptor
d) Radioactive Iodine is the most common therapy

Grave's disease is the **most common cause of hyperthyroidism** and it is caused by autoimmune **IgG** antibodies. Except in children and pregnant patients, **radioactive iodine** is the most common treatment in the US, with 90% cure rate. Medical therapy includes **PTU and methimazole**. **Subtotal thyroidectomy** is indicated for **children, pregnant**, and for patients with compressive symptoms. **Answer B**.

16) 38-year-old female presents to your office complaining of fever and pain on her neck after a recent upper respiratory infection. Physical exam confirmed tenderness, redness, and fluctuance on the left lobe of the thyroid. WBC was mildly elevated and ESR was normal. Appropriate management is:

a) Observation and USG in 2 weeks
b) NSAIDs
c) Incision and drainage
d) FNA

Acute Suppurative thyroiditis usually presents with **fever, fluctuance and elevated WBC**. USG usually localizes the abscess which should undergo **operative I&D**. **Subacute thyroiditis** usually presents with fever, tenderness, sore throat and **elevated ESR**. Treatment is with **NSAIDs** and sometimes steroids. **Answer C**.

17) 71-year-old male presents with a 2.5cm nodule in the right lobe of his thyroid. All of the following pathologic features suggest papillary cancer, **except**:

   a) Intranuclear grooves
   b) Optically clear nuclei
   c) Prominent nucleoli
   d) Multicentric
   e) Amyloid

   Amyloid deposition is a feature of **Medullary thyroid cancer**. **Papillary cancer** is the **most common** thyroid ca, usually **multicentric** (80%), **lymphatic spread**, and rarely metastasizes. **Psammoma bodies** are also are also a feature. **Answer E**.

18) Which of the following is the most common distant site of Papillary thyroid cancer metastasis:

   a) Brain
   b) Liver
   c) Lung
   d) Bone

   Papillary thyroid cancer has the best prognosis (>**90% 10 year survival**) and **rarely metastasizes**. **Children** also have excellent prognosis despite presenting with positive **lymphnode metastasis in ≥50%** of the cases. **Answer C**.

19) 55-year-old male presents with a 1.8cm thyroid nodule and a palpable ipsilateral lymphnode. FNA of the node showed normal thyroid tissue. Which of the following is the most important prognostic factor:

a) Size of the thyroid nodule
b) Presence of metastasis
c) Age
d) Lymphnode status

Age is the most important prognostic factor. **Lymphnode status does not predicts survival** but requires ipsilateral lymphnode dissection if positive. **Answer C**.

20) 40-year-old female was admitted for elective left thyroid lobectomy after FNA of a 1.2cm nodule was indeterminate. Final pathology confirmed Follicular thyroid cancer. Next step in management should be:

a) Iodine therapy after 3 weeks of cytomel
b) Iodine therapy if thyroglobulin levels are elevated
c) Completion thyroidectomy only
d) Completion thyroidectomy with ipsilateral lymphnode dissection

FNA and frozen section are usually **unreliable** to rule out follicular cancer. **Diagnosis** is based on evidence of **capsular and/or vascular invasion**. Rarely metastasizes to lymphnode (**hematogenous spread**), and **lesions > 1cm** should have completion **total thyroidectomy**. **Radioactive iodine for 6 weeks** is recommended for both, follicular and papillary cancer. **Answer C**.

21) 6-year-old girl presents to your office with a palpable thyroid mass and flushing episodes. FNA revealed amyloid. Regarding this condition, all of the following is true, **except**:

a) Most common initial manifestation of MEN II syndrome
b) Flushing and diarrhea are caused by calcitonin secretion
c) Treatment is total thyroidectomy
d) In MEN2b, surgery should be performed by age 2

Treatment of Medullary Thyroid cancer is **Total thyroidectomy and central lymphnode dissection**. MTC arise from **parafollicular C cells** of neural crest origin. Genetic testing should be performed for **RET** proto-oncogene. **MEN2a** should be **operated by age 5** and **MEN2b by age 2. Answer C**.

22) Regarding Hurthle cell cancer, which of the following is false:

a) Routine central node dissection is indicated
b) Considered a variant of Follicular cancer
c) Most are responsive to radioactive iodine therapy
d) Lymphatic spread

Hurthle cell tumors are considered a **subtype of follicular** carcinomas. Differences include: HCT are more often **multifocal**, usually **not responsive RAI**, more likely to **metastasize to local nodes**, and are associated with a higher mortality rate. **Answer C.**

23) Regarding anaplastic thyroid cancer, all of the following is true, **except**:

a) Most are treated with chemoradiation therapy
b) Debulking surgery is not indicated
c) FNA is usually diagnostic
d) Most patients have normal TSH and thyroid hormone levels

Anaplastic thyroid cancers are **undifferentiated** tumors, **extremily aggressive**, and with a disease-specific mortality approaching 100%. **Debulking surgery** (lobectomy) can be used for palliative care and **compressive symproms**.
Answer B.

24) 42-year-old male, s/p total thyroidectomy for a 3cm follicular cancer. Which of the following is the best tumor marker to follow this patient:

a) TSH
b) Thyroxine
c) Thyroglobulin
d) Calcitonin

Thyroglobulin is a glycoprotein **synthesized by neoplastic and normal thyroid tissue**. After **total thyroidectomy**, levels should be **undedectable**, and **if positive, iodine scan** should be obtained. If iodine scan is positive, patient should receive I-131 therapy for microscopic disease.
Answer C.

25) Regarding laryngeal nerve anatomy, which of the following statement is false:

a) RLN is located posterior and medial to superior thyroid artery
b) RLN innervates the vocal cord abductors
c) External branch of the SLN innervates the cricothyroid muscle
d) Unilateral injury to the RLN cause hoarseness

RLN is located next to the **inferior thyroid** artery. Bilateral injury can cause **airway obstruction** due to vocal cords paralysis. **SLN** is located next to the **superior thyroid** vessels and injury may cause **loss of vocal projection**.
Answer A.

26) 26-year-old male with past surgical history of pituitary adenoma resection, presents with kidney stones and a calcium level of 12.6. Which of the following surgical intervention should be performed:

a) Parathyroid adenoma resection
b) Total thyroidectomy with central node dissection
c) Total Parathyroidectomy
d) 3 ½ gland parathyroidectomy

MEN I and IIa syndromes are associated with **parathyorid hyperplasia**. Treatment is **3 ½ gland removal or total parathyroidectomy with autotransplantation**. **Total thyroidectomy** with central node dissection is perfromed for **MTC** at age 5 (MEN IIA) and age 2 (MEN IIB). **Answer D.**

27) 27-year-male was diagnosed with follicular carcinoma of the thyroid involving the inferior pole. During dissection, the surgeon purposely identifies this structure as it **crosses** the recurrent laryngeal nerve before dividing it. What is the structure crossing the RLN:

a) Inferior thyroid artery & branches
b) Superior thyroid artery & branches
c) Vagus nerve
d) hypoglossal nerve

It is known that the inferior thyroid arteries arise from the thyrocervical trunk and travels upward until ending upon the thyroid in its midportion. The inferior thyroid artery crosses the **RLN** and thus should be carefully identified prior to any dividing, as to not cause paralysis to the RLN. Unilateral injury to the RLN would result in **hoarseness**, with bilateral injury causing **airway compromise**. **Answer A.**

28) A patient presents to his PCP with complaints of neck pain. Over the past several weeks, this patient has noticed swelling and pain in the middle of his neck that seems to move when protruding his tongue. He is diagnosed with a congenital anomaly. What is the appropriate treatment for this patient's condition:

a) Thyroidectomy with central neck dissection
b) Thyroidectomy alone
c) En bloc cystectomy alone
d) En bloc cystectomy with partial removal of the hyoid bone

The diagnosis of this patient is a thyroglossal duct cyst, which is considered a common congenital cervical anomaly. During embryology, these cysts usually involute by gestational week 8. Classically, they present as midline masses which moves upward with the protusion of the tongue. Treatment of these cysts involves the **Sistrunk procedure**. This involves en bloc cystectomy with excision of the central hyoid bone. The goal is to eliminate the cyst and decrease recurrence. It is estimated that one percent of these thyrogossal duct cysts can develop **malignancy**. **Infection** is another potential complication. **Answer D.**

29) A middle-aged woman has complaints of dysphagia for the past 3 months, in particular to solid foods. She has experienced no weight loss and her appetite has been unchanged. An oral examination reveals a suspicious mass which appears to extend from the base of her tongue. Treatment of this condition includes:

a) Medical treatment alone with exogenous thyroid hormone
b) Administration of thyroid-stimulating hormone
c) Radioactive iodine ablation alone
d) Surgical excision with hormonal supplementation as necessary

When the median thyroid anlage fails to descend appropriately, patients present with a persistent **lingual thyroid**. A lingual thyroid can become symptomatic, causing obstructive symptoms requiring intervention. The problem with surgical excision is that it may render the patient hypothyroid. Therefore, before any surgical excision takes place, evaluation for existing normal thyroid tissue should be performed. **Answer D.**

30) 30- year-old woman presents with severe flank pain and is diagnosed with nephrolithiasis. Further history-taking reveals patient has had abdominal pain for which previous investigations have been unable to explain the etiology. The surgeon notices in her biochemical profile that her calcium levels are elevated. Being concerned about hyperparathyroidism, he sends a PTH level confirming the diagnosis. What is the next best step:

a) Nuclear medicine imaging
b) CT scan of the cervical region with FNA
c) Minimally invasive surgical resection
d) Observation

This patient has symptomatic hyperparathyroidism. After diagnosis has been confirmed, surgical planning should take place in order to minimize surgical exploration. This should begin with pre operative localization. The 99m Technetium sestamibi is a form of nuclear medicine imaging, which is commonly used to localize, for instance, parathyroid adenomas. In approximately three-fourths of the patients, sestamibi scan identifies abnormal tissue; however it has limitations with small adenomas and /or multiple-gland disease. Some authors recommend ultrasound or CT scan as the initial work up, followed by resection, reserving nuclear studies for cases of "missing gland". It is important to note, most cases of hyperparathyroidism are sporadic (usually adenomas), but some can be familial ie **MEN** syndromes (**hyperplasia**). **Answer A**.

31) A previously healthy 31-year-old male is being evaluated for possible thyroid carcinoma. He initially presented with an enlarging neck mass, progressive hoarseness, and associated palpable cervical adenopathy. Further history-taking reveals he has an uncle who died from thyroid cancer in the past. What percentage of Medullary Thyroid cancers occurs as familial cases:

a) 10%
b) 20%
c) 30%
d) 40%

Of all thyroid malignancies, MTC accounts for 10%, and it is estimated that approximately 20% occurs in the familial setting (ie **MEN-2A**, **MEN-2B**, or familiar non-MEN MTC). These are usually bilateral tumors that occur in the 3rd/4th decade of life. MTC can produce distinct hormones, particularly, **Calcitonin**. Normal calcitonin levels range from 30 to 100 pg/mL. Markedly elevated calcitonin levels found in MTC are usually 1000 pg/mL after provocative testing. **Answer B.**

11. HEAD AND NECK

1) Which of the following nerves supply the cricothyroid muscle:

   a) External laryngeal nerve
   b) Recurrent laryngeal nerve
   c) Hypoglossal nerve
   d) Internal laryngeal nerve

   The cricothyroid muscle is supplied by the external laryngeal nerve (a branch of the superior laryngeal nerve). The **internal branch** of the superior laryngeal nerve is **sensory** to the larynx. The **hypoglossal nerve** is a motor nerve and innervates the **muscles of the tongue**. Almost the entire **larynx** receives its **sensory, parasympathetic**, and skeletal motor nerve supply from branches of the **vagus** nerve. **Answer A.**

2) The left recurrent laryngeal nerve courses around which of the following structure:

   a) Left subclavian artery
   b) Aortic arch
   c) Brachiocephalic artery
   d) Carotid bifurcation

   The **recurrent laryngeal nerve** is a branch of the vagus nerve that supplies the **intrinsic muscles of the larynx**. The left recurrent laryngeal nerve courses around the aortic arch and along the tracheoesophageal groove. The **right recurrent** nerve courses around the **right subclavian** artery with a **more lateral** course than the left. **Injury** can cause **vocal cord paralysis** leading to **dysphonia** and the inability to prevent **aspirations**. **Treatment** consists of **medialization** with Gelfoam. **Answer B.**

3) Which of the following structures does not pass through the parotid gland:

a) Buccal branch of the facial nerve
b) External carotid artery
c) Vestibulocochlear nerve
d) Retromandibular vein

The Facial nerve branches within the parenchyma of the parotid gland. In general, **5 main branches** can be identified: temporal, zygomatic, buccal, mandibular, and cervical. **Answer C.**

4) The borders of the posterior triangle of the neck include all of the following, except:

a) Sternocleidomastoid muscle
b) Trapezius muscle
c) Clavicle
d) Omohyoid muscle

The **posterior triangle** is bounded by the **SCM** anteriorly, the **trapezius** muscle posteriorly, and the **clavicle** inferiorly. It is divided by the omohyoid muscle into an occipital triangle and a supraclavicular triangle and contains the spinal **accessory nerve,** terminal portion of the **subclavian** artery, divisions of the **brachial plexus**, and branches of the thyrocervical trunk. The **anterior triangle** is bounded by the **SCM** posteriorly, the **midline** of the neck anteriorly, and the **mandible** superiorly. It contains the **carotid sheath** and Hypoglossal nerve, and it is subdivided into submental, digastric, carotid, and muscular triangles. **Answer D.**

5) The phrenic nerve can be found running on which muscle of the neck:

a) Anterior scalene
b) Middle scalene
c) Posterior scalene
d) Sternocleidomastoid

The phrenic nerve arises from **C3–5** and courses down in front of the anterior scalene muscle, into the thorax between the subclavian artery and vein. It provides **motor** innervation to the **diaphragm**. **Answer A.**

6) The inferior thyroid artery most commonly arises from which of the following structures:

a) Subclavian Artery
b) External carotid artery
c) Internal carotid artery
d) Thyrocervical trunk

The inferior thyroid artery usually arises from the thyrocervical trunk, but in 10% of individuals it arises directly from the subclavian artery. The **superior thyroid** artery arises from the **external carotid** around the bifurcation of the common carotid artery. **Answer D.**

7) 25 year old male presents with a neck mass that moves upward upon tongue protrusion. What is the most likely location of this thyroglossal duct cyst:

a) Near hyoid bone
b) Base of tongue
c) Mediastinum
d) Near sternocleidomastoid muscle

Most commonly they present as midline masses of the anterior neck. Usually asymptomatic, they may develop **infection** or **thyroid carcinoma**. Some cysts may present more laterally or at the level of the thyroid gland. The vertical motion demonstrates the intimate relation to the hyoid bone. **Sistrunk operation** is the standard method of excision, which includes the center portion of the hyoid bone. **Answer A.**

8) Grave's Disease is an autoimmune condition with antibodies directed against which of the following:

   a) TSH receptors
   b) Parafollicular cells
   c) Thyroglobulin cells
   d) Iodine receptors

   This autoimmune hyperthyroidism is caused by the presence of circulating IgG **autoantibodies** that bind to the G-protein coupled TSH receptor. Management involves 3 modalities, including **pharmacologic** therapy, **RAI** ablation, and **surgical excision**. **Answer A.**

9) What is the embryologic origin of the superior parathyroid glands:

   a) 1st branchial pouch
   b) 2nd branchial pouch
   c) 3rd branchial pouch
   d) 4th branchial pouch

Both the thyroid gland and the superior parathyroid glands derive from the 4th branchial pouch.

Arch and Pouch	Structures
I	Anterior 2/3 of tongue auditory canal, tympanic membrane, middle ear
II	Pharyngeal and palatine tonsils
III	Posterior 1/3 of tongue, Inferior parathyroids, Thymus
IV	**Superior parathyroids; thyroid cartilage**

Answer D.

10) 65 year old male presents with a 3cm papillary cancer of the left thyroid lobe with clinically palpable ipsilateral node. Total thyroidectomy with modified radical neck dissection is scheduled but the patient wants to know which of the following structures will be preserved:

a) Internal jugular vein
b) Internal carotid artery
c) Omohyoid muscle
d) Phrenic nerve

Radical neck dissection is an en bloc removal of all nodal groups between the mandible and the clavicle. MRND spares at least one of the following structures: **SCM, internal jugular vein**, or the **spinal accessory nerve**, while still dissecting Zones I–V. **Answer A.**

11) Which of the following is true regarding carotid body function and nerve supply:

a) Chemoreceptor innervated by Glossopharyngeal and Vagus nerves
b) Chemoreceptor innervated by Glossopharyngeal and Hypoglossal nerves
c) Baroreceptor innervated by Glossopharyngeal and Vagus nerves
d) Baroreceptor innervated by Glossopharyngeal and Hypoglossal nerves

The carotid body is a **chemoreceptor** supplied mainly by the **glossopharyngeal** nerve and fibers from the **vagus** nerve. It is stimulated by **decreased levels of oxygen**, elevated levels of carbon dioxide, and acidosis. Response includes increasing respiratory ventilation. **Answer A.**

12) 55 year old male is completing 1 year after superficial parotidectomy for a mixed tumor, now complaining of sweating around the surgical site during mastication. Most common cause is:

a) Tumor recurrence
b) Aberrant regeneration of parasympathetic fibers
c) Glossopharyngeal nerve injury
d) Hypoglossal nerve injury

Frey syndrome, also known as gustatory sweating, usually presents with **sweating** and **flushing** of the facial skin over the parotid bed **during mastication**. It is thought to be caused by **aberrant regeneration** of cut **parasympathetic fibers**, which leads to innervation of sweat glands and subcutaneous vessels. **Answer B.**

13) 65 year old male presents to your office complaining of a lump over his right mandible for the past 4 months. FNA revealed an acinic cell carcinoma of the parotid gland. Regarding this tumor, all of the following is true, **except**:

   a) 90% occur in the Parotid gland
   b) Most often in women and in the 5th decade
   c) Considered high-grade malignancy
   d) Histologically, there are two cell types

   ACC represents 15% of malignant parotid gland neoplasms. They are typically **low grade malignancies** with two cell types: serous acinar and cells with clear cytoplasm . There are four histologic patterns: papillary, follicular, solid, and microcystic. **Answer C.**

12. CARDIOTHORACIC AND VASCULAR SURGERY

1) Which of the following is true regarding right renal artery anatomy:

   a) Arises from aorta and passes posterior to the IVC/renal vein as it courses to the kidney
   b) Arises from aorta and passes anterior to the IVC/renal vein as it courses to the kidney
   c) Arises from aorta and passes posterior to the IVC and anterior to the renal vein as it courses to the kidney
   d) Arises from aorta and passes anterior to the IVC and posterior to the renal vein as it courses to the kidney

   The right renal artery arises from the aorta and passes posterior to the IVC to the right kidney. The **left renal vein** is longer and passes **anterior the aorta** below the SMA, into the IVC. **Answer A.**

2) Which of the following is the worst preoperative predictor of cardiac complications:

   a) Recent MI
   b) S3
   c) Angina
   d) >5 PVC/min on EKG

   The **Goldman Index** is the best recognized attempt at correlating cardiac symptoms with preoperative complications. It assigns a numeric grade to multiple risk factors. They range from 3-11 points, depending on the symptom.
   11- **uncompensated CHF** (evidenced by elevated CVP/JVD/S3 gallop), 10- recent MI
   7 - > 5 PVC/min on EKG
   7 - non-sinus rhythm or PAC's on EKG
   Answer B.

3) The lesion most likely to require adjunctive revascularization during elective AAA repair is:

a) 50% renal artery stenosis, normotensive
b) Brisk back bleed from Inferior Mesenteric artery
c) 70% stenosis of Celiac artery in asymptomatic patient with normal Superior Mesenteric Artery
d) SMA stenosis and history of right hemicolectomy
e) Prominent Lumbar artery not seen on preoperative angiogram

Criterias for reimplantation include: **back-pressure <40mmHg, SMA stenosis** or inadequate flow to the left colon. It is rarely needed but it should also be considered in patients with **occluded hypogastric arteries,** and in those with **previous colon surgery,** such that normal collaterals have been significantly altered. **Answer D.**

4) A 40 years old male presents to the ER with distal femur fracture after a MVA. On exploration a 1.8 cm segment of the Superficial Femoral artery was bruised and had no palpable pulse over it. Most appropriate management is:

a) Resection with end to end anastomosis
b) Resection with PTFE graft interposition
c) Femoro-Popliteal bypass
d) Suture ligation and fasciotomy

If **less then 2cm**, primary repair should be attempted. Most require an interposition graft. **Reversed saphenous vein** from the uninjured leg should be used whenever possible. The **SFV** should be repaired if possible, and if ligated, calf **fasciotomy** should be performed. **Answer A.**

5) A 65 years old female presented to your clinic with a CT scan of her chest showing a 2 cm peripheral adenocarcinoma involving the right anterior upper lobe. Mediastinoscopy showed no involvement of N2 or N3 nodes. The most appropriate treatment is:

a) Wedge resection
b) Lobectomy
c) Pneumonectomy
d) Chemoradiation

Lung cancer is the **most common cause of cancer-related deaths**. Non–small cell CA (Squamous, Adenocarcinoma, and Large cell) 80%, Small cell 15%, and carcinoids, 5%. **Squamous and small cell** are located **centrally** near the hilum and the incidence of adenoCA is increasing. For **early stage cancer**, **lobectomy** is indicated. Pneumonectomy is rarely indicated and if Cancer is not confirmed, wedge resection should be performed.
Answer B.

6) A 75 year old female with history of atrial fibrillation, presents with acute onset left lower extremity ischemia and demarcation at the midthigh level. Most likely occluded artery is:

a) Aortic bifurcation
b) Internal iliac artery
c) External iliac artery
d) Superficial femoral artery
e) Profunda femoris artery

Occlusion Site	Demarcation Region
Aortic bifurcation	Buttock and proximal thigh
External iliac artery	Midthigh
CFA/Proximal SFA	Calf
Distal SFA / Popliteal Artery	Foot

Answer C.

7) After blunt trauma to the chest, a 50 year old male presented with decreased heart sounds , hypotension and JVD . Which of the following parameters can increase with this condition:

   a) Cardiac Index
   b) MAP
   c) LV stroke work
   d) Coronary artery blood flow
   e) Peripheral vascular resistance

   Cardiac tamponade results in **increased filling pressures** (PA & CVP) and hypotension. In patients with pericardial effusion and hemodynamic compromise, urgent drainage of the pericardium should be performed. **Answer E.**

8) Surgical intervention is indicated for the following asymptomatic 60 year old male:

   a) 4cm AAA
   b) 4.6cm AAA with 3mm growth in 1 year
   c) 2cm common iliac artery aneurysm
   d) 2cm popliteal artery aneurysm
   e) 1cm splenic artery aneurysm

Patients with symptomatic **AAA**, size **> 5.5cm**, and/or **≥0.5 cm increase** in diameter in 6 months should undergo repair. **Splenic** artery aneurysms should be repaired if **> 2cm** or when diagnosed during pregnancy or **child bearing age** (higher risk of rupture). **Popliteal** aneurysms should be repaired because of the **high risk of embolization** and rupture complications. **Answer D.**

9) Which of the following parameters is the most predictive of post-operative pulmonary insufficiency in a patient undergoing pulmonary resection:

   a) RBBB
   b) FEV1 600ml
   c) VC 70 ml/kg
   d) NIF 60 cm

Criteria for lung resection: FEV1 >0.8l (best), DLCO >11, $pCO_2<45$, $pO_2>60$, VO2 max>10 ml/kg/min.

- For pneumonectomy: MVV >55%, $FEV_1>2L$, $FEV_1\%$ >55%;
- For lobectomy MVV >40%, $FEV_1>1$ L, $FEV_1\%$ 40% to 50%;
- For segmental resection MVV >35%, $FEV_1>0.6$ L, $FEV_1\%$ >40%.
  Answer B.

10) 62 year old female had massive pulmonary embolism 5 days after total abdominal colectomy and ileostomy. Duplex revealed unilateral iliofemoral vein thrombosis, and heparinization results in significant improvement. Patient developed gross hematuria followed by shock 2 days later. Best management is cessation of heparin followed by:

   a) Protamine and switch to low molecular weight heparin
   b) Protamine, evacuation of RPH and operative interruption of IVC
   c) Warfarin
   d) IVC filter

One of the indications for IVC interruption is development of **PE with contraindication for anticoagulation**. **Answer D.**

11) 35 year old male was brought by EMS to the ER after being ejected from his car during a MVA. Patient presented with respiratory distress, BP 85/40mmHg, JVD and no breath sounds on the right hemithorax. The pathophysiology of his hemodinamically instability is:

   a) Hypoxemia
   b) Left ventricular outflow obstruction
   c) Compression of the superior and inferior Vena Cava
   d) Increased afterload

Tension pneumothorax develops when air enter the pleural space but doesn't escape; **intrapleural pressure rises**, causing total **collapse of the lung, shift of the mediastinal viscera** to the opposite side, **decreasing venous return** and pre load to the heart. **Answer C.**

12) A 21 year old male, involved in a MVA, presented with respiratory distress, rib fractures and chest x-ray showed massive pneumothorax. After intubation, a 36 Fr chest tube was inserted and massive, persistent air leak was noted. The next step is:

a) Bronchoscopy
b) Decrease the negative pressure on chest tube
c) Thoracotomy
d) Place a double lumen tube and ventilate

Large leaks can contribute to loss of effective tidal volume, resulting in increased VQ mismatch and respiratory acidosis. Bronchoscopy is indicated to rule out **bronchopleural fistula**. **Answer A.**

13) 35 year old male with an incidental finding of a 2cm nodule in the right chest with popcorn calcification. Most likely diagnosis is:

a) Carcinoma
b) Hamartoma
c) Tuberculosis
d) Sarcoidosis

Malignant neoplasms are **larger and grow rapidly**, appear **spiculated**, and with eccentric excavation. **Benign** lesions are **small** (< 1 cm), **stable** (> 2 years), and **calcified.** Incidence of cancer in "coin" lesions is < 10%. Hamartoma is the most common benign adult lung tumor (75%). **Answer B.**

14) Which of the following is true regarding Thoracic duct drainage:

   a) Does not pass through the aortic hiatus
   b) Drains into the right internal jugular vein
   c) Opening into the subclavian vein is protected by valves
   d) Drains the right hemithorax

The thoracic duct is the largest lymphatic channel in the body. It collects lymph from the entire body **except the right hemithorax** and dumps into the junction of the left subclavian vein & left internal jugular vein. **Answer C**.

15) Which one is true regarding vascular graft infections:

   a) Salmonella is frequently isolated
   b) Staphylococcus aureus is most common isolated pathogen overall
   c) Staphylococcus epidermidis is the most common pathogen in late infection
   d) Pseudomonas infection is usually treated with Antibiotic and graft preservation

Most common cause overall - staph epidermidis.
Most common cause of early infection (1 month) - staph aureus
Most common cause of late infection - staph epidermidis

   Answer C.

16) A 61 year old male was referred to your office after routine abdominal USG showed a 5.8cm aortic artery aneurysm. Which one of the following is true regarding his condition:

   a) Caused by decreased proteases activity
   b) Should not be operated at this time
   c) 65% occur between the takeoff of the renal arteries and the aortic bifurcation
   d) Has 40% risk of rupture in 5yr

   Excessive protease activity with **destruction of elastin and collagen** have been implicated in aneurysm formation. Risk factors include **HTN, smoking**, and genetic factors. 90% occur between the renal arteries and the bifurcation. Aproximately 40% AAAs 5.5–6 cm or larger will rupture within 5 years, and 0.5% per year is the rupture rate in AAAs 4–5.4 cm. **Answer D.**

17) The earliest change in atherosclerosis is:

   a) LDL becomes oxidized in blood
   b) Macrophages repair arterial wall causing infl. Reaction
   c) Fatty streak formation
   d) Proliferation of smooth muscle cells

   The correct sequence of events in the process of plaque formation is a)➜ b)➜ c) ➜ d). **Answer A.**

18) 18-year-old male was brought to the ER after sustaining a blunt thoracic injury during a car accident. The most likely site of his thoracic aorta injury is:

   a) Ligamentous Arteriosum
   b) At the root
   c) At the take-off of the left subclavian artery
   d) At the take-off of the Inominate artery

The main risk factor for for this type of injury is **rapid deceleration**. The majority of injuries occur at the aortic isthmus just distal to the left subclavian artery. Second site is at the diaphragm level. Type I injuries (intimal tear) are observed. Type II (hematoma), III (pseudoaneurysm) and IV (rupture) should be repaired. **Answer C.**

19) All of the following are risk factors for atherosclerosis , **except**:

    a) High C-reactive protein levels
    b) Hypoestrogenemia
    c) HIV infection
    d) Hypohomocysteinemia

Hyperhomocysteinemia may reflect deficiency of folate, vitamin B6, or vitamin B12. Homocysteine has primary **atherogenic and prothrombotic** properties. **Answer D.**

20) Which of the following is the most common cause of underlying coronary thrombosis:

    a) Fracture of the fibrous cap
    b) Intraplaque hemorrhage
    c) Proliferation of the vasa vasorum
    d) Plaque erosion producing in situ thrombus

Coronary and carotid plaques have **large lipid cores**, and **plaque rupture** is common. In the femoral artery, superficial plaque erosion more commonly leads to thrombosis. **Answer D.**

21) During Ischemia-Reperfusion injury, firm adherence is mediated by:

    a) P-selectin
    b) PECAM-1
    c) ICAM-1
    d) PSGL-1

Firm neutrophil adherence is modulated by interaction of the β2 integrins with endothelial intercellular adhesion molecule-1 (ICAM-1). **Answer C.**

22) During Ischemia-Reperfusion injury, which of the following proteins is responsible for the first step of the transendothelial migration:

    a) P-selectin
    b) PECAM-1
    c) ICAM-1
    d) PSGL-1

The first step is initiated by increased expression of endothelial P-selectin that interacts with its leukocyte ligand P-selectin. **Answer A.**

23) Which of the following is a pro-inflammatory mediator:

    a) IL-10
    b) IL-4
    c) IL-RA
    d) IL-13
    e) TGF- β

Pro-inflammatory mediators include: IL-1, IL-4, IL-13, MIP-2, TNF, Interferon-γ. **Answer B.**

24) Regarding compartment syndrome, total ischemia causes irreversible nerve damage after:

    a) 30 minutes
    b) 1-2 hours
    c) 4-6 hours
    d) 12 to 24 hours

Clinical signs of compartment syndrome include the **5 P's**: pain, poikilothermia, pallor, paresthesias, and pulselessness. Pulse change is a very late sign. Sensory changes, manifested by paresthesia, may develop after only 30 minutes of ischemia. **Fasciotomy** is the treatment of choice and is indicated when pressure-gradient is > **30mmHg, ischemia** time is **> 6hs** and with associated arterial-venous injuries. **Answer A.**

25) Which of the following is the most common true arterial aneurysm:

   a) AAA
   b) Common Iliac arteries
   c) Femoral arteries
   d) Popliteal arteries

   Pseudoaneurysms of the **femoral artery** are the **most common** of all aneurysms. Infrarenal **AAA** are the **most common** of the **true aneurysms**. **Answer A.**

26) Regarding long term dialysis, patients should be referred for vascular access when their creatinine clearance is less than:

   a) 10 ml/min
   b) 15ml/min
   c) 20ml/min
   d) 25ml/min

   Patient should be referred for permanent dialysis access when their Creatinine clearance is less then 25ml/min. **Answer D.**

27) Which of the following is **not** a common symptom of transient ischemic attack from carotid artery embolism:

    a) Dysarthria
    b) Aphasia
    c) Transient monocular field cuts
    d) Presyncope

    Presyncope is related to hypoperfusion. All other options may occur with carotid artery embolism. **Answer D.**

28) 82- year-old male, history of coronary and carotid artery disease, presented to your office with a duplex USG result showing 80% left carotid artery stenosis. Patient is asymptomatic but meets criteria for elective CABG. Next step should be:

    a) CEA preceding or concurrent with CABG
    b) CABG followed by CEA
    c) Carotid artery stent
    d) Best medical therapy and observation

    After the treatment of their coronary disease patients may become more appropriate candidates to consider intervention for asymptomatic carotid disease. In general, symptomatic disease should be treated first. **Answer B.**

29) Clinical diagnosis of critical limb ischemia is confirmed by:

    a) Ankle pressure < 70mmHg
    b) Toe pressure < 30mmHg
    c) ABI < 0.55
    d) Intermittent claudication

    CLI is characterized by **rest pain, ischemic gangrene**, ankle pressure < 50mmHg and **ABI < 0.4**. The natural history of CLI usually involves progression to amputation unless an intervention is performed. **Answer B.**

30) During carotid artery endarterectomy, the most common injured cranial nerve is:

a) Hypoglossal nerve
b) Ansa cervicalis
c) Marginal mandibular nerve
d) Vagus nerve

Second most common injured nerve is the Hypoglossal.
Answer D.

31) The tibial nerve is located in the:

a) Superficial posterior compartment
b) Deep posterior compartment
c) Anterior compartment
d) Lateral compartment

There are 4 compartments in the calf that need to be released during fasciotomy.

Compartment	Structures
Anterior	Deep Peroneal Nerve, Anterior Tibial Vessels
Lateral	Superficial Peroneal Nerve
Superficial Posterior	Sural Cutaneous Nerve
Deep Posterior	Tibial Nerve, Posterior Tibial vessels

Answer B.

32) Which of the following manifestations is **not** commonly present in patients with post thrombotic syndrome:

a) Ulceration
b) Lower extremity pain
c) Distal ischemia
d) Edema

PTS is caused by **venous outflow obstruction** leading to venous hypertension. Symptoms include edema, pain, hyperpigmentation, and stasis ulceration. **Answer C.**

33) 33 year old male was brought to the emergency department after sustaining a blunt trauma to his neck. Subsequently he developed neurologic changes and a carotid duplex was obtained, confirming right sided carotid dissection. Which of the following is the appropriate initial management:

a) Anticoagulation only
b) Angiogram with balloon angioplasty
c) Angiogram with stent placement
d) Open endarterectomy

Most blunt neck trauma are associated with carotid dissection are successfully managed with anticoagulation only. Open or endovascular interventions are usually reserved for dissections that extend to other vessels. **Answer A.**

34) Regarding Volkmann's ischemic contracture, which of the following is false:

a) Manifests as temporary flexion contracture of the hand
b) Associated with supracondylar fracture
c) Caused by brachial artery thrombosis
d) More common in children

Volkmann's contracture is caused by **brachial artery obstruction** and it is commonly associated with supracondylar fracture. Compartment syndrome may also be the cause, and treatment includes fasciotomy. VC is a **permanent** condition and characterized by ischemic changes of the forearm muscles. **Answer A.**

35) Regarding abdominal aortic aneurysm, which of the following is false:

a) Pararenal aneurysms are localized 1cm below the renal arteries
b) AAA's are defined as a 2.5 fold increase in normal diameter
c) Infrarenal positon in more than 80% of the patients
d) Hypertension increases the risk of rupture

AAA is defined as greater than 3cm dilatation or a **1.5 fold increase** from normal size. Risk factors for rupture include rapid expansion, HTN, family history, HTN and COPD. **Answer B.**

36) 63- year- old female, history of AAA, returns to your office with her annual abdominal CT angiography results. Regarding her condition, which of the following is false:

a) It should be repaired if > 5.5 cm in diameter
b) It should be repaired if annual growth was > 1.0cm
c) If symptomatic, it should be repaired independent of the size or growth
d) Most AAA's are asymptomatic

AAA should be repaired if **symptomatic**, diameter > **5.0cm (female) or 5.5cm (male), or annual growth > 1cm**. Majority is asymptomatic, and risk factors for rupture include smoking, HTN, COPD and female gender. **Answer D.**

37) Which of the following anatomic findings is not a relative contraindication for endovascular repair of abdominal aneurysm:

a) Angulation of 65 degrees
b) Proximal neck of 3mm
c) Common femoral artery diameter of 8mm
d) Distal fixation length of 0.5 cm

Anatomical evaluation is an essential preoperative step before stent placement. Contraindications for EVAR include: **Angulation > 60 degrees, proximal neck length < 1.5cm, distal fixation length < 1.0cm, CFA diameter < 7mm**, and severe calcification/tortuosity on entry sites or landing zones. **Answer C.**

38) 83 year old male with history of HTN, COPD and AAA, presented to the ER complaining of back pain for the past 2 hs. Physical exam revealed hypotension and a pulsatile mass in his abdomen. During his exploratory laparotomy, you notice a large, pulsatile, expanding hematoma in zone 1. After placing a supraceliac clamp and controlling the bleeding, what is the next step:

   a) NGT placement and bilateral iliac arteries dissection
   b) Proximal anastomosis
   c) Heparinization with 80u/Kg followed by arteriotomy
   d) Switching the suprarenal clamp for an infrarenal clamp

   In an unstable patient with rAAA, first step in surgery is to obtain proximal control placing a supraceliac clamp. **NGT** should be in place to assist with the **esophagus identification**. **Supraceliac** cross clamp should be replaced by an infrarenal renal expeditiously, to avoid **renal and splanchnic** circulation **ischemia**. **Answer D.**

39) An 93 year old male returns to your office to schedule his carotid endarterectomy. Upon reviewing his imaging studies you identify a high carotid artery bifurcation. Which of the following is not an appropriate option to facilitate surgical exposure:

   a) Nasotracheal intubation
   b) Posterior mandibular dislocation
   c) Vertical osteotomy of the mandible
   d) Resection of the styloid process

If a high bifurcation is identified preoperatively, **nasotracheal intubation** is the **easiest option** to obtain few mm extra exposure. Intraoperative, the next step should be **division of the posterior belly of the digastrics muscle**. Anterior mandibular dislocation should be used as a last resource. **Answer B.**

40) During conventional CEA, which of the following is the appropriate plane for endarterectomy:

   a) Between anterior and posterior intimal layer
   b) Between intima and media layers
   c) Between anterior and posterior media layers
   d) Between media and adventicia layers

   During conventional CEA, the endarterectomy should start in the CCA between the media and adventicia layers. **Answer B.**

41) A 41 year old male, diabetic, with rest pain performed ABI/PVR studies to evaluate for PAD. His ABI came back as 1.52. Most likely, that result suggests:

   a) Mild peripheral artery disease
   b) Single level stenosis
   c) Calcified distal arteries
   d) Normal exam

   An **ABI above 1.3** should raise suspicion of **stiffened arterial wall** by medial calcinosis, as often occurs in **diabetics**. Because digital arteries are less commonly involved with calcification, toe pressure can be useful when the ABI is falsely elevated. **Answer C.**

42) 65 year old male, POD3 after TEVAR, with purely right sided heart failure. Which of the following is **NOT** an expected hemodynamic finding:

a) Right atrial pressure of 6 mmHg
b) Elevated CVP
c) Normal pulmonary capillary wedge pressure
d) Decreased Cardiac Index
e) Elevated Right ventricle pressure

Righ sided heart failure is associated with elevated right atrial pressure (≥ 10 mmHg) and decreased cardiac index. Diastolic filling pressures in the right atrium and ventricle, and pulmonary capillary wedge pressure, as well as the LV, may be elevated and equalized. **Answer A.**

13. GI HORMONES, ESOPHAGUS AND STOMACH

GI HORMONES

1) Ghrelin is produced in which of the following organs:

a) Brain
b) Stomach
c) Ileum
d) Liver

Ghrelin is most abundant in the **gastric fundus** where it is produced by the endocrine cells P/D1 cells. Its receptor is a member of a G protein-coupled receptor that also includes receptors for motilin and neurotensin. Ghrelin levels **decrease after eating** and evidence indicates that it plays a central role in the neurohormonal **regulation of food intake** and **energy homeostasis. Answer B.**

2) Which of the following is inhibited by the hormone Vasoactive intestinal polypeptide:

a) Gastric acid secretion
b) Pancreas exocrine secretion
c) Pancreas endocrine secretion
d) Vasoconstriction

VIP is an important neurotransmitter throughout the central and peripheral nervous systems. Effects include: **GI secretion and absorption**, bile duct secretion, **smooth muscle relaxation** (including LES and Sphincter of Oddi), and **vasodilatation. Answer D.**

3)   The most potent stimulator of Pancreatic Polypeptide is:

a) Protein
b) Fat
c) Glucose
d) Fatty acids

Protein is the most potent enteral stimulator of PP, followed by fat. PP **inhibits bile secretion, gallbladder contraction**, and **secretion by the exocrine pancreas**. **Answer A.**

4)   Which of the following is the mechanism of action of Sucralfate:

a) Buffering capacity
b) Stimulates pepsin
c) Inhibits mucus production
d) Increases duodenal bicarbonate secretion

In the **presence of gastric acid**, Sucralfate adheres to the gastroduodenal mucosa (reason why it should not be used with PPI's). The drug has almost no buffering capacity, and is believed to provide a **protective barrier**, binding bile salts and inhibiting the actions of pepsin. It also stimulates the production of mucus, **increases mucosal** PGE2 , and increases duodenal bicarbonate secretion. **Answer D**.

5)   Regarding Parietal cells which of the following is true:

a) Secrete HCl and are located in the antrum
b) Secrete pepsinogen and are located in body and fundus
c) Secrete intrinsic factor and are located in the antrum
d) Secrete HCl and are located in body and fundus

G cells are located in the **antrum** and secrete gastrin. **Chief cells** secrete **IF and pepsinogen. Answer D**.

6) Which of the following cells are responsible for the initiation of the migrating motor complex:

a) G cells
b) Interstitial cells of Cajal
c) Parietal cells
d) Chief cells
e) APUD cells

The Interstitial cells of Cajal are also the cells involved in **GIST tumors**. **APUD** stands for amine precursor uptake decarboxylase and is a generic term for a vast group of **endocrine cells** within the gastrointestinal tract. The **antral G cells** secrete gastrin which is responsible for **stimulation of parietal cells** and secretion of acid. G cells are g proteins and act via phospholipase C and PIP. Parietal cells are stimulated by histamine, acetylcholine, and gastrin and release acid. **Chief cells** release **pepsinogen**. **Answer B**.

7) Leptin causes its effects by binding to:

a) G cells
b) Parietal cells
c) D cells
d) Receptors in the arcuate nucleus
e) Receptors in the ileum

Leptin is a hormone that **controls hunger**. It acts to counteract peptide Y and it is produced primarily in adipose tissue. **D cells** make **somatostatin** which universally shuts down the secretion of most enzymes involved in digestion. The **ileum** is responsible for **B12 and bile salt absorption. Answer D**.

8) The histamine receptor on the parietal cell is:

a) A tyrosine kinase
b) An ion channel
c) A G protein
d) Intracellular
e) Associated with facilitated diffusion

The **receptors on the parietal cell** include histamine, acetylcholine, and gastrin. They are **all G protein linked** receptors. **Histamine** uses **adenylate cyclase** to cleave ATP to cAMP while **acetylcholine and gastrin** use **phospholipase C** and PIP. **Tyrosine kinases are transmembrane proteins** and examples include growth factor receptors (VEGFR, EGFR, and FGFR) and RET proto-oncogene. Ion channels are responsible for efflux and influx of ions. **Intracellular receptors include the steroid hormones** which bind to the receptor inside the cell and then enter the nucleus to affect transcription. **Thyroid hormones bind inside the nucleus of cells** and directly affect transcription. **Answer C**.

9) Glucagon-like-polypeptide-1 is produced mainly in the:

a) Brain
b) Stomach
c) Duodenum
d) Ileum
e) Colon

GLP-1 is secreted mainly in the ileum from the L cells and effects **include insulin secretion stimulation and glucagon inhibition** (potential use for treatment of diabetes mellitus).
The **duodenum produces CCK via the I cells, GIP via the K cells, and secretin via the S cells**. The duodenum is also the principal site of **iron and calcium absorption**. **Answer D**.

10)	Omeprazole works by:

a) Blocking receptors on the parietal cell leading to decreased acid production
b) Creating a protective barrier on the stomach lining thus protecting the stomach from acidic contents
c) Decreasing the neural influence on the parietal cell leading to decreased acid production
d) Irreversibly binding to the H/K ATPase leading to decreased acid production
e) Reversibly binding to the H/K ATPase leading to decreased acid production

Omeprazole is a **proton pump inhibitor** and irreversibly binds to the H/K ATPase leading to decreased production of acid. A is the mechanism of histamine blocking drugs such as ranitidine. B is the mechanism of carafate. C occurs when a **vagotomy** is performed. This leads to decreased signaling from the vagus nerve and **less acetylcholine binding to the parietal cell. Calcium leads to increased protein phosphorylation and acid production in the parietal cell,** however, calcium channel blockers are not currently used in the treatment of peptic ulcer disease. **Answer D**.

ESOPHAGUS

1)	The main blood supply to the cervical esophagus comes from the:

a) Inferior thyroid artery
b) Superior thyroid artery
c) Common carotid artery
d) Bronchial arteries

Bronchial arteries supply the **thoracic portion** and the **left gastric artery and inferior phrenic arteries** supply the **abdominal portion. Answer A.**

2) 35 year old male complaining of dysphagia and barium swallow showed a smooth crescent-shaped filling defect surrounded by normal mucosa in the mid-esophagus. Majority can be treated with:

    a) Esophagectomy with 5cm negative margins
    b) Right thoracotomy and simple enucleation
    c) Resection with negative macroscopic margins followed by Imatinib
    d) Balloon dilatation with repeat barium study in 6 months

    Leiomyomas are 50% of the esophageal benign tumors and originate from **smooth muscle**. Dysphagia and pain are the most common complaints. **Biopsy should not be performed** because of an increased risk of mucosal perforation during surgery. Most can be treated with either thoracoscopic or laparoscopic **enucleation. Answer B.**

3) Which of the following is the most common complication of GERD:

    a) Stricture
    b) Barrett's esophagus
    c) Erosive esophagitis
    d) Bleeding

    A **defective LES** is the most common cause of GERD. Esophagitis is the most common complication. **Barret's** is present in ~ **10%** of the patients, **stricture is rare** after acid-reducing therapy era, and **respiratory complications** (asthma, aspiration) may also occur. **Answer C.**

4) 65 year old male with history of chronic gastroesophageal reflux had upper endoscopy performed with biopsies. Pathology confirmed Barrett's esophagus with low grade dysplasia. Management includes:

a) Observation and repeat endoscopy in 6 months
b) Increase PPI dosage and frequent surveillance
c) Endoscopic mucosal ablation
d) Esophagectomy

Barrett esophagus is caused by replacement of the **squamous epithelium by columnar epithelium**. Treatment of BE with **metaplasia** consists of **PPI's or fundoplication**. **Low-grade** dysplasia should be treated for 1–2 months with high doses of PPI's, and if re-biobsy confirms it, **fundoplication** should be considered. **Surveillance** Q6-12 months is indicated. For patients with **high grade** dysplasia (confirmed by 2 pathologists) **esophagectomy** should be considered. Nowadays, endoscopic ablation is another option for BE treatment. **Answer C**.

5) Type III Hiatal hernias are characterized by:

a) Dislocation of the cardia into the posterior mediastinum
b) Dislocation of the fundus into the chest with the cardia in normal position
c) Dislocation of both, the cardia and fundus into the chest
d) Herniation of an additional organ

Hiatal Hernia	Description
Type I (Sliding)	**Most common** type. Dislocation of the cardia into the posterior mediastinum
Type II (Paraesophageal)	Dislocation of the fundus into the chest with the **cardia in normal position**. Usually requires **surgery**.
Type III	Dislocation of the cardia and fundus into the chest
Type IV	Herniation with an **additional organ**

Answer C.

6) 55 year old male was found to have a thin circumferential ring at the distal esophagus, next to the squamocolumnar junction. Patient denies any symptoms. Next step should be:

a) Botulinum toxin injection at 6 months intervals
b) Esophageal dilation
c) Antireflux procedure
d) Observation

Schatzki ring is a narrowing of the lower part of the esophagus caused by a **ring of** mucosal **or muscular tissue** that can cause **difficulty swallowing**. **Symptomatic** Schatzki rings may be treated with esophageal dilatation, using bougie or balloon dilators. **Answer D.**

7) Spontaneous rupture of the esophagus occurs more commonly in the following anatomic position:

a) Left side of the cervical esophagus
b) Left side of the mid-esophagus
c) Left side of the distal esophagus, at the GEJ
d) Right side of the distal esophagus, at the GEJ
e) Both sides equally

Spontaneous esophageal rupture, or **Boerhaave's syndrome**, is caused by **forceful vomiting** or from Valsalva that suddenly **increase intrathoracic pressure**. The perforation in usually occurs in the lower esophagus posteriorly into the left chest. **Surgery** should be performed **within 24h** and consists of **primary repair, with reinforcement** (pleural patch), mediastinal debridement and pleural drainage. If the area is diseased, resection is indicated. **Answer C**.

8) Most commonly, the arterial bleeding from Mallory-Weiss tears will stop with:

a) Ice-water lavage
b) Sengstaken-Blakemore tube placement
c) Endoscopic banding
d) Oversewing of the mucosal tears

The lesion consists of a 1- to 4-cm **longitudinal tear** in the gastric mucosa and submucosa, near the EGJ. **90% of the bleeding stops spontaneously** after ice-water lavage. Next, endoscopic eletrocautery can be attempted, and if bleeding persists, surgery is usually indicated. In addition to blood transfusion, **antiemetic** should be given. **Answer A**.

9) 60 year old male with stage IV esophageal cancer is admitted with complains of severe dysphagia. The mainstay for palliation to improve his symptom includes all of the following, except:

a) Radiation therapy
b) Laser therapy
c) Expandable metallic stent
d) Chemotherapy

Radiation therapy relieves dysphagia in about 50% of patients. Laser therapy in up to 70% and expandable, **metallic stents** are also very useful when **tracheoesophageal fistula** is present. **Answer D.**

10) Esophagectomy should not be performed in which of the following conditions:

a) Barrett's esophagus with high grade dysplasia
b) Scleroderma with "burned out" esophagus
c) Stage II Squamous Carcinoma
d) R0 resection not possible

Surgery is recommended for all esophageal CA patients without metastatic disease who are fit for surgery. **Neoadjuvant chemoradiation** has been shown to improve long-term survival. **Answer D.**

11) Regarding pharyngoesophageal diverticulum, all of the following is true, **except**:

a) Considered a false diverticulum
b) Caused by pulsion forces due to cricopharyngeal muscle dysfunction
c) Killian's triangle is formed by the muscle fibers of the cricopharynfeal muscle and superior constrictor muscle
d) Cricopharyngeal myotomy should be performed for all patients

Zenker's is a **pseudodiverticulum** caused by **dysfunction of the UES**. Located posteriorly **between the cricopharyngeal and lower inferior constrictor muscles**. Patients usually present with **halitosis** and dysphagia, and diagnosis is made with **barium esophagram**. Treatment includes endoscopic or open (for larger ZD) **myotomy** and diverticulectomy/pexy. **Answer C.**

12) Which of the following esophageal diverticula is considered a "true" diverticulum:

a) Pharyngoesophageal
b) Midesophageal
c) Epiphrenic
d) Meckle's

Traction diverticula are considered "true" because they involve **all layers** of the esophageal wall. **ZD and epiphrenic** diverticula are considered **"false"** and associated **motor abnormalities** of the esophagus, UES and LES, respectively. Pathogenesis of **traction** diverticula are **scarring** on the esophageal wall from external inflammatory processes (**tuberculosis**). **Answer B.**

13) 65-year-old male presents to your office complaining of progressive dysphagia and weight loss for the past 5 months. EGD was performed and biopsy confirmed esophageal cancer. Regarding this condition, all of the following is true, **except**:

a) Small tumors can be treated without neoadjuvant therapy
b) Achalasia is one of the risk factors
c) Squamous cell cancer is most common in the lower third of the esophagus
d) EUS is highly sensitive for local staging

Risk factors of esophageal CA include **smoking, ETOH abuse**, achalasia, malnutrition and **Barret's**.
Adenocarcinoma of the esophagus occurs in the **distal third** and **Squamous** in the **proximal** one third.
Neoadjuvant chemoradiation followed by resection is the treatment of choice for T3 or nodal spread CA. Stents can be used as a palliative intervention. **Answer C.**

14) Regarding achalasia, all of the following is true, **except**:

a) Myotomy is the definitive treatment
b) Medical therapy includes forced pneumatic dilatation and Ca channel blockers
c) Parasite infection can be the etiology
d) Caused by absence of ganglion cells in meissner's plexus

Achalasia is a **neurogenic** condition caused by **absence of ganglion cells in Auerbach's** plexus, may be a presentation of a parasitic infection (**Trypanosoma cruzii**) in **Chaga's** disease. Esophagram can show the classic sign **"Bird's Beak"** (narrowing in the distal esophagus) and manometry findings include **failure of the LES to relax** and **uncoordinated peristaltic waves** in the body of the esophagus. Medical therapy also includes **botox injections** and **Heller myotomy** is the definitive treatment.
Answer D.

15) Which of the following is true regarding the vagus nerve and its relation to the esophagus:

a) The right vagus runs anterior and gives off the celiac branches
b) The right vagus runs posterior and gives of the hepatic branches
c) The left vagus runs anterior and gives off hepatic branches
d) The left vagus runs anterior and gives off the criminal nerve of grassi
e) The left and right vagus run anterior

The **left vagus** runs along the **anterior surface** of the esophagus and gives off hepatic branches. The **right vagus** runs along the **posterior surface** of the esophagus and gives off the celiac branches and the **criminal nerve of grassi** (failure to divide this branch leads to persistent high acid output). The mnemonic LHARP can be used (Left hepatic anterior, right posterior). **Answer C**.

16) The internal branch of the superior laryngeal nerve supplies:

a) The mucosa of the larynx
b) The crycothyroid
c) The muscles of the larynx except crycothyroid
d) Tensor tympani
e) The tongue

Internal branch injury results in coughing and an irritating sensation in the throat. **Crycothyroid** is supplied by the **external branch** of the superior laryngeal nerve and causes **voice fatigue**. **Larynx muscles** (except crycothyroid) are supplied by the **recurrent laryngeal**. Paralysis of this nerve results in **hoarseness and paralysis of the vocal cord**. **Tensor tympani** is supplied by the V3 branch of the **trigeminal nerve**, paralysis results in heightened sensation of noise. **Tongue** is supplied by the **hypoglossal nerve**, paralysis results in **deviation towards the side of injury**. **Answer A**.

17) The normal resting tone of the lower esophageal sphincter is:

a) 0 mmHg
b) 20 mmHg
c) 40 mmHg
d) 60 mmHg
e) 80 mmHg

LES: resting tone is **6-26 mmHg, 40 cm from incisors**; total length is about 4 cm (abdominal length about 2cm). **UES**: resting tone about **60 mmHg**, located 15 cm from incisors, and about 5 cm in length. **Answer B**.

18) Normal lower esophageal tone combined with high amplitude contractions of long duration is consistent with which of the following esophageal motility disorders:

a) Achalasia
b) Hypertensive lower esophageal sphincter
c) Diffuse esophageal spasm
d) Nutcracker esophagus
e) These are normal findings

Disorder	LES	Esopha-gram	Amplit-ude pressure	Peristalsis
Achalasia	Failure to relax	Bird beak/dil-ated esoph-agus	Decreased	None
Hyper LES	High	Distal obstruct-ion	Normal	Normal
DES	WNL/ slightly elevate d	Corkscre w	Normal	None
Nut-cracker	Norma l	Normal progress-ion	Very high	Hyper-tensive
Sclero-derma	Low	"foamy" or air	low	none

Answer D.

19) A 72 year old female patient presents to your clinic with complaints of halitosis and old regurgitated food on her pillow when she awakens in the morning. This pathologic process is a result of:

a) Hypertensive cricopharyngeus muscle
b) A traction diverticulum
c) A diverticulum near the base of the diaphragm
d) Herniation of the stomach into the thoracic cavity
e) Frequent retching and vomiting

Zenker's occurs secondary to a **hypertensive cricopharyngeus** muscle which causes a diverticular outpouching in the upper esophagus. Treatment is via diverticulectomy with myotomy. If **large** enough, it can be **obliterated endoscopically** with the use of a stapling device. Pexy is also an option. Diverticuli can be divided into true, false, traction, and pulsion. Pulsion diverticuli typically are false diverticuli and occur as a result of increased pressure. Examples include epiphrenic and Zenkers. **Epiphrenic** are frequently accompanied by esophageal **motility problems**. Herniation of the stomach into the thorax is encountered with hiatal and diaphragmatic hernias. Hiatal hernias are divided into type I or sliding, type II or paraesophageal, type III which is combined type I and II, and type IV where additional abdominal contents herniate such as colon and spleen. Frequent retching and vomiting can cause Mallory Weiss tears. These frequently heal on their own but if treatment is needed, endoscopic or open oversewing usually controls the bleeding. **Answer A.**

20) The surgical approach for mid esophageal lesions is typically via:

a) Median sternotomy
b) Cervical incision
c) Right thoracic approach
d) Left thoracic approach
e) Transabodminal approach

The esophagus courses to the **left then to right and then back to the left as it traverses the thoracic cavity**. For this reason surgical approaches in the chest correspond to this anatomic snaking. Lesions in the **upper esophagus** are approached by a **cervical incision or left thorax**, and lesions in the **lower esophagus** are attacked via **left thorax** and abdominal approach. There are **three areas of physiologic narrowing** of the esophagus. They occur at the **cricopharyngeus** in the upper esophagus, at the level of **T4 in the mid esophagus** near the carina, and at the **lower esophagus** as it exits the diaphragm. **Answer C**.

21) The esophagus is unique from the other parts of the gastrointestinal tract in that:

a) It lacks peristaltic activity
b) There is a circular muscle layer
c) There is no serosal covering
d) It is partly under voluntary control
e) It has a sphincter

The esophagus lacks serosa layer. It is in close contact with the tissues of the neck and has an **adventitial layer instead**. The esophagus does have a circular muscle layer, is partly under voluntary control, and does have physiologic sphincters but these features are not unique to the esophagus. **Answer C**.

STOMACH AND DUODENUM

1) Blood supply to the duodenum is derived from:

a) Gastroduodenal and Right Gastroepiploic arteries
b) Gastroduodenal and superior mesenteric arteries
c) Left gastroepiploic and Common Hepatic arteries
d) Pancreaticoduodenal and right gastroepiploic arteries

The Duodenum is supplied by the **Superior and Inferior Pancreaticoduodenal** arteries, branches of the GDA (which is a branch of the common hepatic artery) and SMA respectively. The GDA terminates by dividing into the right gastroepiploic and anterior superior pancreaticoduodenal arteries. The **common circulation** between the duodenum and **head of the pancreas** is the main reason why both are usually resected together. **Answer B.**

2) Following Parietal cell vagotomy, expected outcome includes:

   a) Normal gastric emptying and frequent episodes of diarrhea
   b) Decreased gastric emptying and infrequent episodes of diarrhea
   c) Increased gastric emptying and infrequent episodes of diarrhea
   d) Normal gastric emptying and infrequent episodes of diarrhea

   In PCV, **antral innervation is spared** (Nerves of Latarjet) and a drainage procedure is not indicated. **Dumping and diarrhea** are much **less** than after proximal vagotomies. Usually indicated for **intractable duodenal ulcers**. **Answer D.**

3) Which of the following gastric ulcer procedures have higher recurrence rates:

   a) Truncal Vagotomy, antrectomy, and Billroth I reconstruction
   b) Truncal Vagotomy, antrectomy, and Billroth II reconstruciton
   c) Proximal Gastric vagotomy
   d) Truncal Vagotomy with piloroplasty

Incidence of dumping and post vagotomy diarrhea are much higher after truncal vagotomies.

GU Procedure	Mortality	Recurrence
PCV	<0.5%	10%
TV with antrectomy	2%	2%
TV with piloroplasty	1%	8%

Answer A.

4) Which of the following is not a typical characteristic of Gastrinoma:

a) Usually present as microadenomas
b) Most APUDomas are Non-B islet cell ca. of the pancreas
c) 30 % are associated with MEN-1
d) Positive Alfa-HCG is suggestive of malignancy

10% are microadenomas and more than 50% are Islet cell tumor. Common presentation includes severe/refractory PUD and diarrhea. **Hypergastrenemia with acid hypersecretion** is highly suggestive of Gastrinoma, and very high gastrin levels with the presence of alfa-HCG suggest malignancy. **Somatostatin-receptor scintigraphy** is extremely sensitive for **localization** and treatment is medical (acid reducing therapy) and surgical (**enucleation** or resection). **Answer A.**

5) Type I Gastric ulcers are characterized by all of the following, except:

a) Normal gastric acid output
b) Most common type of gastric ulcer
c) Antral gastritis is rare
d) Located in the lesser curvature

Gastric Ulcer	Acid Output	Location/Features
Type I	Low	Lesser curvature, near the incisura. Most common type, usually associated with antral gastritis and H. Pylori
Type II	High	Prepyloric and associated with duodenal ulcers
Type III	High	Prepyloric
Type IV	Low	High on the lesser curve, near GEJ
Type V	Normal	May occur anywhere; Associated with chronic use of NSAIDs.

Answer C.

6) Which endoscopic finding has the highest recurrence rate of upper GI bleed:

   a) Clot at the base of the ulcer
   b) Diffuse bleeding
   c) Visible vessel at the ulcer
   d) Pulsatile bleeding

   The higher risk of rebleeding, in descending order is: Active arterial bleeding →non-bleeding visible vessel →adherent clot →oozing without visible vessel → flat spot → clean ulcer base. **Answer D.**

7) Regarding Gastric lymphoma, which of the following statement is false:

   a) Majority are B-cell non-Hodgkin Lymphoma
   b) MALT lymphoma should be treated with antibiotics
   c) Splenectomy should be performed in High grade lymphoma
   d) Chemotherapy is the treatment of choice for Low grade lymphoma

The stomach is the **most common extranodal site** of lymphoma (NHL). 70–80% of patients with **MALToma** will have a complete regression with antibiotic eradication of *H. pylori*. First line therapy of **lymphomas**are usually with **chemotherapy**, but **surgical resection** can be considered for **early stages** or complications. The spleen should be removed only if it is also involved with the tumor. **Answer C.**

8) Regarding Gastrointestinal tumors, all of the following is true, **except**:

a) Imatinib is used for disseminated disease
b) Metastasectomy improves outcome
c) Radiosensitive
d) Bleeding is the most common presentation

GISTs originate from the interstitial **cell of Cajal** and are characterized by the expression of the **CD117 antigen**, which is part of the **KIT** transmembrane receptor tyrosine kinase. Main prognostic determinants are tumor **size (>10cm), mitotic rate (>5/50 hpf), and tumor location (small intestine)**. Generally, **1-2 cm margin is recommended** and lymphnode dissection is unnecessary. GISTs are highly sensitive to Imatinib (**Gleevec**), but **resistant to radiation** therapy. **Chemotherapy** should be **used if disease progresses**. **Answer C.**

9) Early gastric cancers are defined by invasion of the following layers:

a) Mucosa only
b) Mucosa and Submucosa
c) Muscularis propria
d) Serosa

Early gastric cancer is defined as adenocarcinoma limited to the mucosa and submucosa, **regardless of lymph node status**. Cure rate after resection is approximately 95%. Risk factors include **blood type A, smoking, chronic/atrophic gastritis**, HNPCC, **H. Pylory**, pernicious anemia, and **nitrosamines**. Histologic types are **diffuse or intestinal**. **Answer B.**

10) Gastric cancer involving the cardia should be resected with:

a) Subtotal gastrectomy with omentectomy and Bilroth I
b) Antrectomy with Bilroth II
c) Esophagogastrectomy
d) Total gastrectomy with splenectomy

Due to the propensity of gastric CA to spread in the submucosa, at least **5cm gross margins** should be obtained. The standard operation is **subtotal gastrectomy**. Total gastrectomy confers no additional survival benefit with higher perioperative morbidity and mortality.It is indicated only to obtain a R0 resection in proximal tumors. Oncologic resection entails tumor resection, lymphnode removal, en block resection if needed, and negative margins. **Answer A.**

11) Which of the following is the most common site of gastric cancer:

a) Antrum
b) Lesser curvature
c) Cardia
d) Linitis plastica

Linitis plastica involves the **entire stomach** and occurs in 10% of gastric CA patients. Majority occurs in the lesser curve, followed by the cardia. **Answer B.**

12) Regarding post-gastrectomy complications, which of the following is false:

a) Marginal ulcer is an ulcer on the gastric side of the gastrojejunostomy
b) Diarrhea occurs in 10% of those patients
c) Gastroparesis is associated with Roux-en-Y procedure
d) Bile reflux gastritis after BII can be treated with Braun enteroenterostomy

Post gastrectomy complications include:
Dumping (early and late) from **hyperosmolar food and reactive hypoglycemia**. If refractory, treatment is conversion to a Roux-en-Y gastric bypass;
Marginal ulcer is a **jejunal ulcer** caused by **incomplete vagotomy** (diagnosed by Sham feeding test), **retained antrum** (radionuclide scan) or **Gastrinoma** (secretin test). Treatment includes H.Pylori eradication, vagotomy, and gastrectomy;
Bypassing the duodenum may cause deficiency of Ca, Iron, Vitamins B12, A, D, E, K, and folate;
Bile reflux gastritis may occur after **pyloric resection**, causing N/V (bilious) and epigastric pain. Besides Braun procedure, treatment also includes **conversion from BI or BII to Roux-en-Y**.
Diarrhea is common and caused by bile malabsorption, **bacterial overgrowth**, and **rapid gastric emptying**.
Answer A.

13) You perform and EGD on a 54 year old male with history of GERD who takes PPI's, and find a 1.5 cm polyp in the antrum. You remove the polyp endoscopically and send the lesion to pathology. The report identifies the lesion as an adenomatous polyp. What is the next best step:

a) Stop the PPI and obtain CT abdomen and pelvis
b) Repeat EGD in one year
c) Wedge gastrectomy
d) Bilroth II with 5 cm margins

There are multiple types of polyps in the stomach just as there are in other parts of the GI tract. **Adenomatous polyps <2cm** in size can be **endoscopically removed** and a **repeat EGD** can be performed. It is reasonable to **look for synchronous lesions** in the remainder of the GI tract because nearly a third of patients will have adenocarcinoma in the GI tract. The **most common types** of polyps are **fundic gland, adenomatous, and hyperplastic. Fundic gland** polyps (FGP) are most common and occur in the setting of **PPI** usage. They are multiple, small polyps which harbor nearly no malignant potential. FGP's are also associated with **FAP** and should be suspected in young patients. **Hyperplastic** polyps occur frequently in **atrophic gastritis and H. pylori**, are found in the antrum, and harbor **low malignant potential. Answer C**.

14) Following Ivor Lewis esophagectomy, the main blood supply to the stomach is via:

a) Right gastric
b) Left gastric
c) Right gastroepiploic
d) Left gastroepiploic
e) Short gastrics

The **left gastric** artery is a branch of the **celiac trunk** and **supplies the lesser curvature**. The **right gastric** artery comes off the **hepatic artery** and also supplies the **lesser curvature**. The **left gastroepiploic** artery is a branch of the **splenic artery** supplying the **greater curvature**. The **right gastroepiploic** artery arises from the **gastroduodenal artery** and also supplies the **greater curvature. Answer C.**

15) Which of the following is not a critical step when performing laparoscopic Nissen fundoplication:

a) Obtaining 2 – 3 cm of intraabdominal esophagus length
b) Creating a loose 360 degree wrap
c) Division of the short gastric vessels
d) Anterior closure of the crural defect
e) Dissection of the lesser omentum

All of the above are critical steps of a Nissen fundoplication, however, the **crural defect is best repaired posteriorly**. This can be accomplished with or without a mesh. **Answer D**.

14. HEPATOBILIARY SYSTEM

LIVER

1) Neoplastic cyst of the liver are characterized by all of the following, except:

   a) Mucinous fluid
   b) Elevated CA 19-9
   c) Low density fluid
   d) Multilocular

   Neoplastic cysts have irregular wall, elevated CEA/CA 19-9 and higher density/mucinous fluid. **Simple Cyst**: Almost all simple cysts do not usually require treatment. However, cyst more than 4 cm may require frequent monitoring to assure that they are stable. **Cystadenomas**: The preferred treatment for cystadenomas is resection, (15 % Malignancy rate). Removal of the cyst can be accomplished by enucleating it from the surrounding liver. If cystadenocarcinoma is suspected, treatment should consist of a formal liver resection. **Answer C.**

2) Treatment options for Hydatid cyst includes all of the following , except:

   a) Albendazole
   b) Percutaneous aspiration for centrally located cysts
   c) Pericystectomy
   d) Liver transplantation

Echinococcosis is diagnosed by a combination of imaging and serology. Though surgery remains his gold standard for cystic echinococcosis treatment,there have been a number of studies that suggest that PAIR **(Percutaneous aspiration, injection and** reaspiration) with chemotherapy is more effective than surgery in terms of disease recurrence, and morbidity and mortality If surgery is contraindicated, PAIR should be performed. **Answer D.**

3) Which of the following is false regarding Cavernous hemangioma:

a) Hypointense lesion on T-1 weighted MRI
b) Peripheral to centripetal enhancement of the lesion on CT scan
c) Surgical options include enucleation or liver resection
d) Main blood supply is from the venous system

Cavernous hemangiomas are the most common benign liver tumors. Large hemangiomas can occasionally cause symptoms as a result of compression of adjacent organs or intermittent thrombosis, which results in expansion of the lesion. Surgery may be considered an option **only** if the patient is symptomatic. The risk of rupture, embolization is low as a result the size alone should not be an indication of surgery. **Answer D.**

4) Which of the following is false regarding Focal Nodular Hyperplasia:

a) Stimulated by oral contraceptives
b) Majority of lesions are solitary and has central scar
c) Hypodense lesion on pre contrast CT and hypointense on T1 weighted MRI
d) Sulfur colloid scan are positive

Focal nodular hyperplasia (FNH) is a benign tumour of the liver (hepatic tumour), which is the second most prevalent tumour of the liver (the first is hepatic hemangioma) Focal nodular hyperplasia's most recognizable gross feature is a central stellate scar. They have Kupffer cells as a result they are **positive** on colloid scan compared to Hepatic Adenoma which are negative on Colloid scan. Also tagged RBC scan would be **negative** (positive in hemangiomas). **Answer A.**

5) Which of the following is false regarding Hepatic adenomas:

a) Strongly associated with oral contraceptives
b) Most lesions are solitary
c) Lesions are hypointense on T1 weighted MRI
d) Surgical resection should be performed

Oral contraceptives, anabolic androgens, and glycogen storage disease are strongly associated for **Hepatic adenomas**. CT scan shows hypervascular lesion during the arterial phase and **negative** uptake on Sulfur colloid uptake. Also tagged RBC scan would be **negative** (positive in hemangiomas). For tumor < 4 cm, cessation of contraception, steroid is recommended for tumor > 4 cm, and if patient does not have any steroid use. **Answer C.**

6) Which of the following is not part of the MELD (Model for End-stage Liver disease) score in prioritizing liver transplant patients:

a) Creatinine
b) Serum Albumin
c) Bilirubin
d) INR

MELD is a validated chronic liver disease severity scoring system that uses a patient's laboratory values for **serum bilirubin, serum creatinine, and the international normalized ratio** for prothrombin time (INR) to predict survival. In patients with chronic liver disease, an increasing MELD score is associated with increasing severity of hepatic dysfunction and three-month mortality risk. MELD = 3.8[Ln serum bilirubin (mg/dL)] + 11.2[Ln INR] + 9.6[Ln serum creatinine (mg/dL)] + 6.4 (Very frequently asked). **Answer B**.

7) During preoperative transplant evaluation, preserved Liver function can be confirmed by the following test:

a) Gama-GT
b) Creatinine Clearance
c) Indocyanine green clearance
d) Bilirubin

Indocyanine & Normal Portal pressure is the best predictor of Liver function. Indocyanine. Portal venous pressure is the blood pressure in the hepatic portal vein, and is normally between 5-10 mmHg. **Wedge hepatic venous pressure (WHVP)** is used to estimate the portal venous pressure by reflecting not the actual hepatic portal vein pressure but the **hepatic** sinusoidal **pressure**. It is determined by wedging a catheter in a hepatic vein, to occlude it, and then measuring the pressure of proximal static blood (which is reflective of pressure in the sinusoids). **Answer C.**

8) 45 year old male present to the ER complaining of a 1 week history of fever, nausea, anorexia and RUQ pain. CT was obtained and showed air-fluid level in segment IV of the Liver. Most common etiology is:

a) Cryptogenic
b) Pylephlebitis, from appendicitis or diverticulitis
c) Biliary ductal system
d) Trauma

Biliary tract disease such as gallstones or malignant obstruction is present in 40 to 60 percent of **liver abscess**. Additional source include hematogenous spread. Most common organism is Gram negative and antibiotics with percutaneous drainage are usually indicated. Treatment of **Uniloculated pyogenic liver abscess** should include percutaneous drainage and antibiotic therapy. However, **multiloculated liver abscess**, septic patient usually requires surgical resection. **Answer C.**

9) 69 year old male, on propranolol, with a history of cirrhosis and Portal venous pressure of 10mmHg was admitted for recurrent variceal bleeding after endoscopic banding. Next step in management should be:

a) TIPS
b) Esophageal devascularization
c) Splenorrenal shunt
d) Liver transplant

Two Endoscopic modalities are currently the definitive treatment of choice for active variceal hemorrhage: **Sclerotherapy and Esophageal band ligation**. Balloon tamponade is an effective way to achieve short-term hemostasis if endoscopic therapy fails and TIPS not readily available. **Transjugular intrahepatic portosystemic shunting** (TIPS) is indicated in patients in whom hemorrhage from esophageal varices cannot be controlled or in whom bleeding recurs despite combined pharmacological and endoscopic therapy. Medical therapy and endoscopic treatment control most of these bleeding, but for recurrent bleeding and normal liver function, TIPS is indicated. **Answer A.**

10) Which of the following is the most effective therapy for refractory ascites:

a) Large volume paracentesis
b) Peritoneovenous shunt
c) Portosystemic shunt
d) Liver transplantation

Patients with **diuretic-resistant ascites** undergo serial paracentesis and follow a sodium-restricted diet (2 g/day) rather than undergo TIPS as initial therapy. Liver transplantation is the only definitive therapeutic option but the management of ascites is an important issue until transplantation. **Answer D.**

11) Which of the following is the treatment for amoebic liver abscess:

a) Percutaneous drainage
b) Metronidazole treatment
c) Percutaneous aspiration, injection and reaspiration
d) Hypotonic saline

Patient with **amoebic liver abscess** present with fever and abdominal pain. Diagnosis is achieved by ELISA and radiology. Treatment is **with metronidazole** 50 mg tid for 7 to 10 days and is successful in 95% of cases. **CT of the liver** is used to follow up after initial treatment. Aspiration of the abscess is rarely needed for multiloculated abscesses that do not respond to medical therapy, abscesses that appear to be superinfected, and abscesses of the left lobe of the liver that may rupture into the pericardium. **Answer B.**

BILIARY SYSTEM

1) 61 year old male, asymptomatic, was found to have gallstones in surveillance abdominal USG for post operative AAA. Cholecystectomy should not be performed if:

   a) Gallstone > 2cm
   b) Polyps > 1.5cm
   c) Calcified gallbladder
   d) Life expectancy < 20 years

The important symptom of g**allstones** is biliary colic. Biliary colic is a severe pain in the right upper quadrant radiating to the back and right shoulder, which may be accompanied by nausea. Despite its name, the pain is usually steady and not colicky. Pain is worse after ingestion of fatty foods. Prophylactic cholecystectomy is **not** indicated in most patients with asymptomatic gallstones. **Indication for prophylactic cholecystectomy** includes patients who are at increased risk for gallbladder carcinoma or gallstone complications, in whom prophylactic cholecystectomy or incidental cholecystectomy at the time of another abdominal operation can be considered. Patients with diabetes mellitus have an increased risk of complications, but risk of cholecystectomy does not outweigh prophylactic cholecystectomy. **Answer D.**

2) 42 year old female presents to the ER complaining of a 5 day history of fever, nausea and right upper quadrant pain. Bilirubin was 6, RUQ USG showed large gallstone in the cystic duct, CBD of 9mm and no CBD stones. Most likely diagnosis:

a) Pyogenic abscess
b) Pylephlebitis
c) Mirizzi's syndrome
d) Cholangiocarcinoma

Mirizzi syndrome is caused by extrinsic compression of common hepatic duct obstruction by an   an impacted stone in the cystic duct or Hartmann's pouch of the gallbladder. Open cholecystectomy remains the standard of care for Mirizzi syndrome with compression of the common duct facilitating the removal of the causal factors: the inflamed gallbladder and the impacted stone. Although laparoscopic surgery may be possible in some patients with favourable anatomy, for patients with a fistula, or erosion into the common duct, the choice of repair depends on the extent of the damage to the common duct. **Answer C.**

3) During cholecystectomy, in order to obtain the "critical view of safety", the surgeon should:

a) Perform cholangiography in selected patients
b) Dissect the Cystic duct-CBD junction
c) Dissect the peritoneal attachments and retract the infundibulum anteriorly
d) Retract the gallbladder superiorly and the infundibulum laterally

After **critical view** is obtained, the cystic duct and artery are the only two structures entering the gallbladder and they can be safely clipped. **Answer D.**

4) The test of choice to rule out cystic or bile duct leak should be:

a) HIDA scan
b) ERCP
c) MRCP
d) RUQ USG

ERCP and HIDA can both identify **post choleycystectomy leaks,** but HIDA is less invasive and should be attempted 1st. If there is delayed presentation, the biliary anatomy should be defined using percutaneous cholangiography, and the bile leak should be controlled with percutaneous biliary stents and intra abdominal drains. Repair is ideally performed six to eight weeks after control of the leak and after intraabdominal sepsis is resolved. Hepaticojejunostomy rather than end-to-end anastomosis represents the best option for repair for most common bile duct injuries. **Answer A.**

5) 25 year old female, 6 weeks pregnant, presented to the ER complaining of nausea, vomiting, fever, and RUQ pain. WBC was 14 and RUQ USG revealed gallstones and small amount of pericholecystic fluid. Management should be:

a) Laparoscopic cholecystectomy
b) Antibiotics and conservative management
c) Biliary drainage
d) ERCP and sphincterotomy

Acute cholecystitis is associated with RUQ pain, fever, and elevated WBC due to gallbladder inflammation caused by cystic duct obstruction. **Pregnancy** decreases gallbladder motility and increases the cholesterol saturation of bile. Cholecystectomy is recommended for recurrent attacks and is safest during the **2nd** or early **3rd** trimester. **Answer A.**

6) 56 year old female presented to the ER complaining of fever, nausea and RUQ pain for the past 24hs. Vital signs were: BP 90/60mmHg; Pulse 105; Temperature 39C. RUQ USG showed gallstones and CBD measuring 10 mm. Shortly after patient developed confusion. Next step in management should be:

a) IV antibiotics and PTC
b) IV antibiotics, Blood Cultures, transfer to the SICU for observation
c) Intravenous hydration and antibiotics
d) Laparoscopic cholecystectomy

Acute cholangitis is caused primarily by bacterial infection where the organisms typically ascend from the duodenum. The common predisposing factor for acute cholangitis is biliary obstruction and stasis secondary to biliary calculi or benign stricture. The classic **triad of Charcot** — fever, right upper quadrant pain, and jaundice — occurs in only 50 to 75 percent of patients with acute cholangitis. In ases of severe cholangitis (Raynaud's pentad: Charcot's + Confusion and hypotension), initial therapy should be IV fluid administration and IV antibiotics followed by biliary decompression. If available, ERCP should be attempted before PTC. **Answer A.**

7) Most common cause of bile duct injury is:

a) Inadequate inferior retraction of the gallbladder
b) Excessive cephalad retraction
c) Short cystic duct
d) Presence of inflammation

Complete transection of the common bile duct is the most frequent biliary injury, and is difficult to manage . This "classic" injury occurs when too much traction of cystic duct lines it paralled to the common bile duct and the common bile duct is mistaken for the cystic duct, resulting in clipping and division of the common duct, which is then resected with the gallbladder. Bile duct injuries are classified as **Bismuth and Strasberg classification. Answer B**.

Types	Strasberg-Bismuth Classification
A	Ducts of Lushka or cystic duct leaks
B	Partial occlusion of the biliary tree
C	Transection of aberrant right hepatic ducts
D	Lateral injuries to major bile ducts
E	Common hepatic or CBD division

8) Which of the following describes a Type III choledocal cyst:

a) Dilatation of the common hepatic or bile duct
b) Supraduodenum diverticulum of the common hepatic or bile duct
c) Choledococele
d) Multiple cysts involving intra and extra biliary tract

Choledochal cyst	Features	Treatment
Type I	Saccular or fusiform dilatation of a portion or entire common bile duct	Surgical excision of the cyst with hepatico Jejunostomy roux-en-Y anastomosis to the biliary duct
Type II	Isolated Diverticulum off CBD	Cyst excised and primary closure of choledochotomy
Type III	Arise from dilatation of duodenal portion of CBD	Transduodenal approach with marsupialization or cyst excision.
Type IV	Dilation of both intrahepatic and extrahepatic biliary system.	Partial liver resection vs hepatioc jejunostomy vs liver transplant
Type V (Caroli's disease)	Cystic dilatation of intra hepatic biliary ducts	Partial liver resection vs hepatioc jejunostomy vs liver transplant

Answer C.

9) 69 year old female, post operative day 3 status post laparoscopic cholecystectomy, has no complaints at this time. Final pathology report showed gallbladder tumor invading the subserosal layer. Management includes:

a) Radiation followed by Chemotherapy
b) Chemotherapy only
c) Liver bed excision with Segment IV and V resection
d) Liver resection with periportal, peripancreatic and celiac nodes removal.

Chronic gallbladder inflammation , Porcelain gallbladder , **Gallbladder polyp > 10 mm**, Primary sclerosing cholangitis are risk factors for Gallbladder carcinoma.

Gallbladder adenocarcinoma	Treatment
T1 (Mucosa +lamina propria)	Cholecystectomy
T 2 (Muscularis propria)	Wedge resection of segement IV and V with 2-3 cm margin with portal trial lymphadenectomy
T3/4 (beyond muscle and resectable)	Formal resection of segment IV and V, Portal triad lymph nodes excision and CBD excision with hepatico-jejunostomy.

Answer D.

10) 70 year old female with significant cardiac history and multiple abdominal surgeries, presented to the ER complaining of nausea, vomiting, obstipation and hypotension for the past 24hs. Abd X ray showed pneumobilia and air fluid levels. Management should be:

a) IV hydration, antibiotics, NGT placement and observation in the ICU
b) ERCP and sphincterotomy
c) Enterolithotomy
d) Enterolithotomy and cholecystectomy

Chronic inflammation between gallbladder and 2nd portion of duodenum from chronic cholecystitis can lead to gallstones being released in small bowel causing Gallstones ileus. Big Stones can cause Small bowel obstruction commonly obstructing at **Terminal ileum**. Air in biliary tree with dilated loops of small bowel is classic finding on AXR. Treatment of Gallstone ileus involves NPO, NGT, and hydration. Laparotomy with removal of stone with longitudinal enterotomy proximal to obstruction is recommended. If patient is not **stable**, gallbladder duodenal fistula can be left alone. If patient is **stable,** choleycystectomy, resection of fistula and closure of the duodenotomy is recommended. **Answer A**.

15. PANCREAS AND SPLEEN

PANCREAS

1) Which of the following is not part of the Ranson's criteria in biliary pancreatitis:

a) Age > 70
b) WBC > 18000 mm3
c) Serum glucose > 200 mg/dl
d) Serum LDH > 400 (U/L)

At Admission	After 48 hours
Age in years > 55 years	Serum calcium < 2.0 mmol/L (< 8.0 mg/dL)
White blood cell count > 16000 cells/mm³	White blood cell count > 16000 cells/mm³
Blood glucose > 200 mg/dL	Oxygen (hypoxemia P$_{O2}$ < 60 mmHg)
Serum AST > 250 IU/L	BUN increased by 1.8 or more mmol/L (5 or more mg/dL) after IV fluid hydration
Serum LDH > 350 IU/L	Base deficit (negative base excess) > 4 mEq/L
Score 3-4: 15 % mortality Score 5-6: 40% mortality Score 7-8: 100 % mortality	Sequestration of fluid > 6L

Answer A.

2) 42 year old male with recurrent episodes of acute pancreatitis. ERCP demonstrated failure of fusion of the dorsal and ventral pancreatic ducts. Treatment include:

a) Distal pancreatectomy
b) Minor papilla sphincterotomy
c) Major papilla sphincterotomy
d) Puestow procedure

Pancrease divisum is failed fusion of pancreatic ducts, Duct of Wirsung and Duct of Santorini. Duct of Wirsung is normally opens in major papilla. As a result of the non fusion, duct of Wirsung is a short duct on ERCP and Duct of Santorini appears as a long duct. Recurrent pancreatitis may result from duct of Santorini stenosis. Treatment is ERCP or open duodenotomy with **Sphincteroplasty of minor papilla i.e. Duct of Santorini. Answer B.**

3) A pH probe is advanced into the duodenum and sequential pH measurements are taken from the pancreatic ductal secretion. Administration of which of the following substances will lead to a rise in the pH values:

a) Cholecystokinin
b) Somatostatin
c) Glucagon
d) Secretin
e) Gastrin

Many hormones affect pancreatic exocrine and endocrine function. Secretin stimulates the release of HCO_3- from the pancreatic ductal cells. CCK stimulates the pancreatic enzymatic release. Gastrin stimulates stomach acid production, while somatostatin inhibits pancreatic exocrine and endocrine function. **Answer D.**

4) 64 year old male, history of alcohol abuse and recent admission for recurrent pancreatitis, comes to your office for a routine visit .Patient denies any symptoms but a CT scan showed a 5cm pancreatic pseudocyst. Best management is:

a) Cystgastrostomy
b) Endoscopic drainage
c) Observation
d) Percutaneous drainage

In the past, surgeons used to indicate intervention for pseudocysts greater than 6 cm or longer than 6 weeks. Currrently, the indications are pseudocysts complicating acute or chronic pancreatitis who are **symptomatic** or **infected**. The size can be monitored and symptoms(pain, fever, jaundice) should be investigated. Transpapillary stenting for communicating and small pseudocyst, is recommended. **Cystenterostomy** is ideal for large and symptomatic pseudocysts when there is close apposition to the GI tract. **Answer C.**

5) Which of the following is the most common cause of acute pancreatitis in the United States is:

a) Gallstones
b) Alcohol
c) Hyperlipidemia
d) Drug related

The most common **causes** of acute pancreatitis are **alcohol use** and **choledocholithiasis** The most effective decision aids at admission include APACHE-II, CRP, and BISAP criteria. Apache II score > 8 predicts Sever Acute Pancreatitis(SAP). Procalcitonin is the most promising new marker being evaluated for prediction of SAP. BUN> 25, Altered Mental Status, SIRS, Age > 60, Pleural effusion **(BISAP).** > 3 of above predicts SAP. In mild disease, nutrition can be maintained through a diet as tolerated. In severe disease, early enteral nutrition has been shown to be beneficial. If enteral nutrition is poorly tolerated because of ileus, TPN should be considered. **Prophylactic antibiotic** is not recommended and is considered in severe pancreatitis with suspicion of infection. **Indications** for intervention include infected necrosis, sterile necrosis with prolonged failure, and abdominal compartment syndrome.
Answer A.

6) 56 year old male with history of ETOH abuse presented to the ER complaining of epigastric pain, nausea, vomiting for 2 days after heavy drinking. Amylase and lipase were elevated. Next step in management is:

a) NGT placement and IV antibiotics
b) ERCP
c) CT scan of the abd and pelvis
d) IV fluids and observation

Mainstay of acute pancreatitis treatment is **supportive**, with adequate nutrition, pain control and correcting electrolytes imbalance. If tolerated, **Nasojejunal tube feeds** should be started early to improve nutrition status and prevent translocation of bacteria.IV antibiotics are only indicated for infected necrosis. **Answer D.**

7) 77 year old male was admitted with hematemesis and after endoscopic intervention was found to have isolated gastric varices. Best management is:

a) Endoscopic banding
b) TIPS
c) Splenectomy
d) Vasopressin

The most common cause of isolated **splenic vein thrombosis** is chronic pancreatitis caused by perivenous inflammation. The incidence of splenic vein thrombosis is high upto 45 % with chronic pancreatitis, but most patients with SVT remain asymptomatic. Splenectomy effectively eliminates the collateral outflow and is the treatment of choice. TIPS are used for patients with concomitant portal hypertension or as a bridge to liver transplant. **Answer C.**

8) 58 year old male presented to the ER with hemodynamic instability and upper GI bleed. Upper endoscopy visualized blood coming out from the papilla. Best treatment is:

a) Cholecystectomy and biliary drainage
b) ERCP , sphincterotomy and stent placement
c) Angioembolization
d) Whipple procedure

Hemobilia can occur following liver injuries, radiologic interventions. When patients have upper gastrointestinal bleeding following liver injury or biliary tract intervention, hemobilia must be ruled out. The classic triad of hemobilia is **right upper quadrant pain, jaundice, and upper gastrointestinal bleeding**, although this may not be present in all patients. Appropriate management of these patients is with **hepatic angiography and embolization**. Rarely, operative intervention may be required for debridement or resection of large intrahepatic pseudoaneurysms. **Answer C.**

9) 69 year old male with history of ETOH abuse, heavy tobacco use and hyperlipidemia was found to have a pancreatic mass. Most important risk factor for adenocarcinoma is:

a) Benzene exposure
b) Hyperlipidemia
c) Tobacco use
d) ETOH abuse

Smoking and obesity are risk factors for the development of **pancreatic ductal adenocarcinoma**; industrial asbestos exposure, experimental radon exposure, alcohol abuse, and diabetes appear to be less clearly associated. Surgical resection via **pancreaticoduodenectomy** (PD) is the only potentially curative therapy; such resection improves the overall 5 year survival rate to 15% to 25%. Only a minority (20% to 30%) of patients at the time of diagnosis are candidates for surgical resection because of the presence of locally advanced disease, distant metastases, or significant medical comorbidities. The surgical resection rates are very low for periampullary malignancies since they are the most aggressive tumor in this area. **Answer C.**

10) 50 year old male on post operative day 7 after laparoscopic splenectomy, was found to have a 5x5cm fluid collection in the LUQ. After percutaneous drainage, the fluid was found to have elevated amylase. Next step in management is:

a) ERCP and stent placement
b) Distal pancreatectomy
c) Conservative management
d) Tagged RBC scan

Majority of pancreatic fistulas heals spontaneously with nutritional support and supportive care. Low output **pancreatic fistula** is defined as output less than 200 mL/day, and most will resolve spontaneously if adequate drainage without obstruction is established. High output lateral fistulae (greater than 700 mL/day) are rare..Early ERCP with sphincterotomy and/or stenting may help with resolution. Use of subcutaneous injections of somatostatin analog to lower the incidence of pancreatic fistula after Whipple resections and after distal pancreatectomy is recommended but Randomized controlled trials refute the benefits. Prospective data using this agent in large numbers of patients are lacking. **Answer C.**

11) Which of the following endocrine tumor is associated with diabetes and gallstones:

a) VIPoma
b) Somatostatinoma
c) Glucagonoma
d) Insulinoma

Somatostatinomas usually presents with abdominal pain and weight loss.Tumors within the pancreas present with the triad of **DM, Diarrhea with steatorrhea, and Gallstones**. DM and Gallstones result from decreased release of insulin and CCK, respectively. Steatorrhea is caused by inhibition of pancreatic enzyme and bicarbonate secretion. **VIPoma** is associated with achloridria, watery diarrhea and hypokalemia; **Glucagonoma** causes DM and necrolytic migratoryerythema; **Insulinoma** is the most common pancreatic endocrine tumor. Somatostatin receptor scintigraphy (SRS) is very sensitive for pancreatic neuroendocrine tumors. Intraoperative USG is also very useful to help localize these tumors. **Debulking** of the metastatic tumors improves survival rates and symptoms. **Streptozosin and 5-FU** are used as adjuvant therapy. **Answer B.**

12) A 42 year-old male presents with complaints of dizziness, diaphoresis and palpitations that improves with a meal. On laboratory work-up he is found to have elevated C-peptide levels and fasting blood glucose of 35mg/dL. Preoperative imaging studies have failed to identify a pancreatic mass. Selective arterial stimulation with which of the following substances could help localize the lesion:

a) Ocreotide
b) Calcium Gluconate
c) IGF-1
d) Potassium chloride
e) Secretin

Arterial calcium stimulation with hepatic venous sampling involves selective injection of calcium gluconate into the GDA, splenic, and SMA arteries. **Calcium stimulates the release of insulin from beta cells (insulinomas or nesidioblastosis), but not normal beta cells**. **Answer B.**

13) A 53-year-old male is hospitalized with severe gallstone pancreatitis. CT scan of the abdomen revealed a necrosis of approximately 50% of his pancreas. He has been treated with aggressive medical management for the past 7 days and despite therapy he has persistent leukocytosis, rising temperatures, and hemodynamic instability. Blood cultures as well as other cultures have failed to grow organisms. What is the next step in management of this patient:

a) Laparoscopic pancreatic debridement
b) Endoscopic transgastric pancreas debridement
c) CT guided aspiration
d) CT guided drainage
e) Prophylactic Imipenem

CT-guided percutaneous aspiration with Gram's stain and culture is recommended to rule out infected pancreatic necrosis. **Sterile necrosis** does not usually require antibiotics, but if there are signs of infection, percutaneous aspiration is recommended. Surgical debridement should be performed with infected necrosis is confirmed. **Answer C.**

14) A 41-year-old female is diagnosed with acute pancreatitis. Which of the following, if present on admission, is indicative of more severe disease:

a) Glucose 180
b) PaO2 65mmHg
c) AST 350
d) LDH 280
e) Calcium 7.5

Ranson's criteria is one of the earliest scoring systems to assess the severity of pancreatitis. Factors such as Age >55, WBC >16, Glucose >200, AST >250, LDH >350 are assessed on admission and Hct decrease of 10, BUN increase of 5, Calcium <8, PaO2 <60, base deficit >4 and fluid sequestration >6L are assessed after 48 hours of admission. Although it continues to be used clinically, its ability to accurately predict the severity of pancreatitis is being questioned. **Answer C.**

15) A patient with idiopathic recurrent pancreatitis is found on ERCP to have independent dorsal and ventral pancreatic ducts that have failed to fuse. Optimal treatment of this patient is aimed at:

a) Stenting major papilla
b) Surgical re-anastomosis of the ducts
c) Transecting minor papilla sphincter
d) Transecting and repairing major papilla sphincter
e) Pancreatic head resection

Pancreatic divisum is the most common pancreatic anomaly present in up to 7% of the general population. This condition arises from the embryological failure to fuse between the ventral and dorsal pancreatic ducts. Most patients are asymptomatic, but a small percentage goes on to develop symptoms. The therapeutic goal is aimed at addressing the minor papilla by either endoscopic or surgical sphincterotomy and/or sphincteroplasty in order to facilitate drainage of dorsal pancreas. **Answer C.**

16) 56- year-old female presents with abdominal epigastric pain radiating to her back. Serum amylase 800, lipase 12500, bilirubin 3.2, AST 215, ALP 250. CT scan reveals gallstones, no biliary ductal dilation and the presence of peri-pancreatic inflammation as well as a 3mm common bile duct stone. You make the diagnosis of gallstone pancreatitis and treat this patient conservatively initially. Within the following 3 days her liver function test normalized and her clinical exam is much more improved. Next step in management is:

   a) ERCP with sphincterotomy and stone extraction
   b) Laparoscopic cholecystectomy with intraoperative cholangiogram
   c) Laparoscopic cholecystectomy with common bile duct exploration
   d) Laparoscopic cholecystectomy alone
   e) Discharge patient home and bring as outpatient in 6 weeks for elective laparoscopic cholecystectomy

ERCP should be performed within 72 hours in **gallstone pancreatitis** with high suspicion of persistent bile duct stones. Cholecystectomy should be performed after recovery and during same admission. If the suspicion of persistent CBD stones is low, laparoscopic cholecystectomy with intraoperative cholangiography is preferable to avoid the morbidity associated with ERCP. Laparoscopic or Open cholecystectomy with common bile duct exploration are reserved for patients in which you have identified CBD stones and have failed or are not candidates for endoscopic therapy. **Answer B.**

17) 37 year-old female underwent laparoscopic splenectomy for ITP. She presents 7 days post-op with an abdominal fluid collection. CT guided drainage was performed and fluid analysis showed an amylase level of 110,000. The catheter output is approximately 350cc per day. You manage the patient with conservative measures. Which of the following initial therapies may help reduce the drain output:

a) Subcutaneous ocreotide injection
b) Laparoscopic selective closed-suction drain placement
c) Sclerosing agent inside drain
d) Intravenous secretin and pancreatic polypeptide infusion
e) ERCP with pancreatic stenting

Pancreatic fistula is the result of leakage of pancreatic secretions from disrupted ducts. 80% of pancreatic fistulas close spontaneously with conservative measure. Subcutaneous ocreotide injections may be helpful at decreasing fistula output in patients with high output (>200cc/day) and allow for electrolyte correction and preventing further skin breakdown from drainage. However, ocreotide does not decrease the rate of fistula closure. Endoscopic treatment is a reasonable option once initial conservative management has failed. **Answer A.**

18) Which of the following characteristics indicate unresectability of a pancreatic neoplasm:

a) 3 cm lesion in head infiltrating ampulla
b) 1.5 mm direct invasion of tumor into SMA
c) A single 1cm lesion confined to right lower lobe of the lung
d) 2 peri-pancreatic enlarged lymph nodes
e) 5cm lesion involving tail and infiltrating close to splenic hilum

NCCN guidelines define unresectability as:
Head of pancreas lesions: Greater than 180 degrees SMA encasement, any celiac abutment, unreconstructable SMV/portal vein occlusion, Aortic invasion or encasement
Body: SMA or celiac encasement greater than 180 degrees, unreconstructable SMV/portal vein occlusion, aortic invasion.
Tail: SMA or celiac encasement greater than 180 degrees.
For all sites: Distant metastases, Metastases to lymph nodes beyond the field of resection.
A minimal infiltration into major visceral vessels such as the SMA is now considered borderline resectable whenever reconstruction is feasible. **Answer C.**

19) 19- year-old female complains of epigastric pain. She has been taking proton-pump inhibitors without clinical improvement for several weeks. Upper gastrointestinal endoscopy reveals multiple duodenal ulcers and gastric ulcers. You are concerned about a gastrinoma. Which of the following studies would best help you localize the tumor:

a) Secretin stimulation test
b) Abdominal CT scan
c) Somatostatin receptor scintigraphy with SPECT
d) Transabdominal ultrasound
e) MRI

Gastrinomas are usually located within the gastrinoma triangle, but they can occur anywhere. The test of choice for localization is a somatostatin receptor scintigraphy (SRS). By itself it detects approximately 85% of gastrinomas including lesions <1 cm. The combination with single **photon emission CT (SPECT) and EUS** increases its accuracy to about 90%. With newer technological advances in CT and MRI it remains a question whether detection accuracy will improve with these modalities in the future specially at detecting smaller lesions. **Answer C.**

20) Six weeks after an episode of acute pancreatitis a 45 year-old male was incidentally found to have a peri-pancreatic simple fluid collection approximately 8 cms on CT scan. He denies any complaints of abdominal pain, fever or early satiety. What would you recommend for this patient:

a) Laparoscopic cystjejunostomy
b) Conservative management
c) Laparoscopic cystgastrostomy
d) CT guided percutaneous drainage
e) EUS drainage

Pancreatic pseudocysts are common in patients with acute and chronic pancreatitis as well as trauma. Many of them are asymptomatic and resolves spontaneously. A watchful waiting approach is now indicated for asymptomatic pseudocysts that are not enlarging. Surgical management with internal drainage is still the gold standard for those who are good operative candidates and meet the indications. **Answer B.**

21) Which of the following pancreas neuroendocrine tumors is not well localized by somatostatin scintigraphy:

a) Insulinoma
b) Glucagonoma
c) Gastrinoma
d) VIPoma

Somatostatin receptor scintigraphy (SRS), has a high sensitivity in most pancreatic neuroendocrine tumors but is a poor method for insulinomas since insulinomas fail to express somatostainoma receptor. EUS can also be useful, but it is operator dependendent and may be less sensitive for lesions in the tail. Tumors may also be biopsied, making the diagnosis unequivocal and eliminating false-positive results. **Intraoperative ultrasound (IOUS)** is the most sensitive method of detection and localization. More invasive preoperative localization procedures, such as calcium angiogram and portal venous sampling are less commonly used. Surgical exploration with IOUS is indicated when the diagnosis of insulinoma has been made biochemically, even if preoperative localization was unsuccessfull. **Answer A.**

22) 72- year-old female presents with abdominal epigastric pain radiating to her back. Serum amylase 800, lipase 12500, bilirubin 3.2, AST 215, ALP 250. U/S shows no gallstones, no biliary ductal dilation and the presence of peri-pancreatic inflammation as well as 6mm pancreatic duct dilation. You make the diagnosis of pancreatitis and treat this patient conservatively initially. Within the following 3 days her pancreatic function test normalized and her clinical exam is improved. A CT scan is obtained and a mass is identified in the head of pancreas. All of the following are true, **except**:

a) ERCP with bare metal stent has long term higher patency over plastic stent
b) Chemoradiotherapy will improve the survival of unresectable periampullary tumor
c) Gastrojejunostomy is indicated for duodenal obstruction
d) Preoperative chemoradiotherapy may improve respectability of borderline resectable tumor

Pancreaticoduodenectomy (PD) is the operation of choice for patients with periampullary malignancy. In patients who are seen initially with obstructive jaundice, endoscopic retrograde cholangiography (ERC) serves both a diagnostic and therapeutic function. Cholangiography can exclude certain benign causes, such as choledocholithiasis, and it can help identify the presence of a distal CBD stricture. Patients with cholangitis, intractable pruritis, or major nutritional deficiency may benefit from **preoperative stenting.** Locally advanced disease limits the chances for a successful margin-negative resection, thus patients in this group are typically offered **neoadjuvant chemoradiation** to downstage the tumor. **Answer B.**

23) Which of the following is not a common presentation of Glucagonoma:

a) Diabetes
b) Skin rash
c) Mass in the tail of the Pancreas
d) Jaundice

Glucagonoma is characterized by a pancreatic mass, new onset Diabetes and a typical rash (**necrolytic migratory erythema**). Patients do not present with jaundice because it is usually located in the tail of the pancreas. **Answer D.**

24) 42 year old male presented to the ER complaining of watery diarrhea for the past 4 weeks. Lab work revealed a WBC 14, Na 135 and K 2.5. Patient was severely dehydrated and CT showed a 2 cm mass in the tail of the pancreas. Most likely diagnosis is:

a) Glucagonoma
b) Somatostatinoma
c) VIPoma
d) Gastrinoma

VIPoma usually presents with watery diarrhea, hypokalemia and achlorhydria (**WDHA**). Medical management includes **somatostatin** analogues and surgical treatment consists of **tumor debulking**, hepatic artery embolization and RFA for liver metastasis. **Answer C.**

25) 52 year old male was diagnosed with an endocrine tumor of the pancreas. Most likely diagnosis is:

   a) Glucagonoma
   b) Insulinoma
   c) Gastrinoma
   d) VIPoma

   Typical presentation of the most common endocrine pancreatic tumor is the **Whipple triad**, which consists of a serum glucose level < 50mg/dl, symptomatic fasting hypoglycemia and improved symptoms after glucose administration. **Answer B.**

26) 26 year old nurse presented to the ER with a third episode of symptomatic hypoglycemia this year. Her lab work revealed high levels of C peptide and her insulin to C peptide ratio was 0.5. Most likely diagnosis is:

   a) Insulinoma
   b) Juvenile Diabetes
   c) Factitious hypoglycemia
   d) Glucagonoma

   Factitious hypoglycemia or self-administration of insulin is suggested by **low C peptide level** and insulin to C peptide ratio > 1. Treatment depends on size and location. Most insulinomas are benign and can be treated by **enucleation. Answer A.**

27) Which of the following is not characteristic of somatostatinoma:

 a) Cholelithiasis
 b) Hyperchlorhydria
 c) Steatorrhea
 d) Type II DM

Most common symptoms are abdominal pain and weight loss. Tumors localized within the pancreas sometimes cause the 3 classic findings: **diabetes, cholelithiasis, and diarrhea** with steatorrhea. **Hypochlorhydria** may also occur. If the primary tumor is not visualized on cross sectional imaging, EUS, or **somatostatin receptor scintigraphy** may be used. Surgical resection is the treatment of choice. **Answer B.**

SPLEEN

1) Which of the following is the most common indication for splenectomy:

 a) Hereditary spherocytosis
 b) Thrombotic thrombocytopenic purpura
 c) Trauma
 d) Immune thrombocytopenic purpura

ITP is the most common non traumatic indication for splenectomy and is managed first with steroids then immunoglobulin. Splenectomy is indicated in patients whose medical therapy has failed, in those who recurr, or when prolonged steroid use causes side effects. If platelet transfusion is required perioperatively for bleeding or counts below $10,000/mm^3$, transfusion should be held until the splenic artery is ligated. **TTP:** First-line treatment is with daily plasmapheresis and FFP transfusions. Splenectomy in TTP is reserved for patients who have frequent relapses. **Answer C**.

2) 24 year old male undergoing elective laparoscopic splenectomy for ITP , post splenectomy sepsis prevention is best obtained by:

a) IV penicillin 24hs before and after the procedure
b) Vaccination against encapsulated organisms 24hs before followed by PO penicillin post operative
c) PO penicillin before any invasive procedures
d) Vaccination 2 weeks before the procedure

Risk factors for **OPSI** include age (chidren at 5% vs. adults at 0.9%), splenectomy for a hematologic disorder, and history of immunosuppressant therapy. The risk for OPSI is highest in the first 2 years after surgery but does carry a lifelong risk. OPSI has a reported fatality rate of 50%. *Streptococcus pneumoniae, Neisseria meningitides,* **and** *Haemophilus influenzae* B account for most of the severe infections.   Patients typically come in with an upper respiratory infection that rapidly proceeds to sepsis and multisystem organ failure. A high index of suspicion for OPSI is required, and early and aggressive treatment with broad-spectrum antibiotics and supportive measures can be life saving.Patients should be immunized against streptococcus pneumonia (most common), meningococcus and H. influenza 2 weeks after trauma cases and 2 weeks before elective cases. Most common organism involved in OPSI is **Strep pneumonia. Answer D.**

3) Where is the most common site of an accessory spleen:

a) Tail of pancreas
b) Splenic hylum
c) Superior pole of the left kidney
d) Small bowel

Accessory spleen is present in up to 20% of the population. Over 80% of accessory spleens are found in the region of the splenic hilum and vascular pedicle. Post splenectomy, patients with an accessory spleen will have an absence of Howell-Jolley bodies, Heinz bodies, and target cells and may require reexploration for accessory spleens or selective embolization. **Answer B.**

4) 24 year old female, 2 weeks post laparoscopic splenectomy, presented to the ER complaining of fatigue. Blood tests showed WBC 18000, Hb 16, Platelets 1.000.000 and Heinz bodies. Most likely diagnosis:

   a) Normal post splenectomy changes
   b) Acute leukemia
   c) Accessory spleen
   d) Lymphoma with bone marrow invasion

After splenectomy, expected changes include **increased RBCs, WBCs, Platelets and nuclear remnants**. Aspirin is the treatment of choice for Platelets greater than 1 million. As splenectomy causes an increased risk of sepsis due to encapsulated organisms (such as S. pneumoniae and Haemophilus influenzae) the patient should receive the pneumococcal conjugate vaccine, Hib vaccine, and the meningococcal vaccine. These bacteria often cause a sore throat under normal circumstances but after splenectomy, when infecting bacteria cannot be adequately opsonized, severe sepsis occurs. Splenectomy patients typically have Howell-Jolly bodies and less commonly Heinz bodies in their blood smears, target cells. **Answer A.**

5) 45 year old male presented to the ER complaining of fever, anorexia and weight loss for the past 2 weeks. CT scan of the abd demonstrated splenic abscess. Best management is:

a) IV antibiotics, nutritional support and admission to ICU
b) IV antibiotics and percutaneous drainage
c) Splenectomy
d) Surgical drainage

Streptococcus is the most common organism causing **splenic abscess** and splenectomy is the treatment of choice. Initial medical treatment for splenic abscesses remains intravenous antibiotics, beginning with broad-spectrum coverage and then tailored to a culture-specific regimen. Percutaneous aspirates can be useful in guiding antibiotic therapy. **Percutaneous splenic abscess drainage** can be safe and effective in selected patients with small **uniloculated abscess**. However Failure rates are high. In multiloculated abscesses, Splenectomy can provide definitive treatment for splenic abscess. **Answer C.**

6) 16 year old male was brought to the ER after falling from his bicycle. Blood pressure was 100/60mmHg and Pulse 95. CT scan of the abdomen showed a Grade IV splenic laceration. Next step should be:

a) Observation
b) Partial Splenectomy
c) Splenectomy
d) Angioembolization

Blunt mechanisms are more common in splenic injury. CT findings include hypodensity, intraparenchymal or subcapsular hematoma, contrast blush, or hemoperitoneum. Splenic injury is graded I through V depending upon the extent and depth of splenic hematoma and/or laceration. Per ATLS protocol, hemodynamically **unstable** patients with a positive FAST exam or DPL require surgical exploration. For **stable** patients with low grade (I to III) injuries, non operative initial management is suggested. For stable patients with **active** contrast extravasation, **splenic embolization** is suggested. **Answer A.**

7) 37 year old male with thrombotic thrombocytopenic purpura should be initially treated with:

a) Steroids
b) Plasmapheresis
c) Cyclophosphamide
d) Splenectomy

Thrombotic Thrombocytopenic purpura is characterized by profound thrombotic event with low platelets, mental status change, renal failure, fever and microangiopathic hemolytic anemia. Deficiency of **ADAMTS13** which is responsible for cleavage of vWF results in uninhibited thrombosis. MCC of death is intracerebral hemorrhage and acute renal failure. First-line treatment is with daily plasmapheresis and fresh frozen plasma (FFP) transfusions. Most patients will respond to therapy. Splenectomy in TTP is reserved for patients with frequent relapses. **Answer B.**

8) 80 year old male with history of anorexia, weight loss and ascites was admitted for diagnostic paracentesis. Fluid was rich in proteins and white colored. Most common cause is:

a) Splenic cancer
b) Pancreatic ascites
c) Lymphoma
d) Cirrhosis

Common causes of **chylous ascites** includes **lymphoma**, ovarian cancer, pancreatic ca, lymphangiomyomatosis, carcinoid, retroperitoneal sarcomas. Abdominal paracentesis is the most important diagnostic tool in evaluating and managing patients with ascites.

Color	Milky, cloudy
TG level	>200 mg/dl
Cell count	>500 (lymphocyte predominant)
Total protein	>3.0

In patients in whom the cause cannot be found or for those who do not respond to treatment of the underlying condition, a high protein and low fat diet with medium-chain triglycerides (MCT) is recommended. In patients with pancreatic ascites, who do not respond to conservative management, treatment with octreotide (50 micrograms given subcutaneously three times daily for two consecutive weeks) and ERCP for pancreatic duct stenting is recommended. **Answer C.**

9) Which of the following requires splenectomy in most of the patients:

a) Chronic lymphocytic leukemia (CLL)
b) Acute lymphcocyti leukemia
c) Hairy cell leukemia with neutropenia
d) Sickle cell anemia

Splenectomy confer survival advantage in patient with **CLL** with anemia and thrombocytopenia, Hairy cell leukemia. No survival advantage is noted in patients with CLL without anemia/Thrombocytopenia. Prior to era of CT scan, Splenectomy was commonly indicated for staging Hodgkin's lymphoma. **Portal venous/ SMV thorombosis** is ture complication common after splenectomy done for hematologic disorders. **Answer A.**

10) Which of the following is the most common cause of non traumatic splenic rupture worldwide:

a) Mononucleosis
b) Malignancy
c) Malaria
d) ITP

In the US, **Mononucleosis** is the most common cause of non traumatic splenic rupture. Spontaneous splenic rupture is a rare but potentially fatal complication of infectious mononucleosis. Abdominal pain is uncommon in infectious mononucleosis, and splenic rupture should be strongly considered whenever abdominal pain occurs. In developing countries, **Malaria** is the most common cause of splenic rupture. **Answer C.**

11) 41 year old male with RUQ pain was found to have cirrhosis with 2 cm mass in the periphery of segment VI of liver. Patient has history of alcoholic cirrhosis and Upper GI bleed 3 months ago. On further work up of the mass revealed isolated hepatocellular carcinoma without any metastasis. CT scan revealed splenomegaly. Which of the following is contraindication to laparoscopic splenectomy:

a) Malignancy
b) Autoimmune thrombocytopenia
c) Portal hypertension
d) Platelet count 50K

Malignancy, thrombocytopenia (platelet > 20 K), ITP are not a contraindication for laparoscopic splenectomy. However, Laparoscopic splenectomy is **contraindicated** in patient with portal hypertension due to the risk of massive bleeding. **Answer C.**

16. SMALL BOWEL

1) Which of the following portions of the Duodenum are located in the retroperitoneum:

   a) 1st and 2nd
   b) 2nd and 3rd
   c) 2nd and 4th
   d) 3rd and 4th

   Retroperitoneal segments are the 2nd and 3rd. Vascular supply includes Superior Pancreaticoduodenal artery (anterior and Posterior) branch of gastroduodenal artery, Inferior pancreaticoduodenal artery (anterior and posterior) branch of SMA. Inferior pancreaticoduodenal branch is the first branch of SMA. **Wilkie disease** (SMA syndrome) occurs in lean, thin patients or weight loss post gastric bypass where the partial obstruction of 3rd porion of duodenum occurs by SMA. Treatment includes increasing dietary content to improve weight or duodenojejunostomy. **Answer B.**

2) Which of the following is mainly absorbed in the Duodenum:

   a) Vitamin B12 and Folate
   b) Bile salts
   c) Iron and Calcium
   d) NaCl and water

B12 and folate are absorbed in the terminal ileum, Bile salts in the ileum and most of NaCl and water are absorbed in the jejunum. The most common deficiency after gastric bypass surgery is vitamin B_{12}, folate, zinc, iron, copper, calcium, and vitamin D and can lead to secondary problems, such as osteoporosis, Wernicke encephalopathy, anemia, and peripheral neuropathy.

Common nutritional deficiencies in patients who have had gastric bypass surgery	
Vitamin B12, Folate	Megaloblastic anemia, peripheral neuropathy
Vitamin D, Calcium	Osteoporosis
Copper	Pancytopenia, Ataxia
Iron	Anemia

Answer C.

3) During which of the following phase of the Migrating motor complex gallbladder contraction occurs:

a) Phase I
b) Phase II
c) Phase III
d) Phase IV

Phase I is the resting phase, in II gallbladder contraction and acceleration occurs, Phase III is the Peristaltic phase (stimulated by motilin) and phase IV is the deceleration phase. This process starts in stomach and progresses through the small intestine over a perior of **2 hours**. It is **stops with meals. Answer B.**

4) Which of the following is the main source of fuel for enterocytes:

a) Short chain Fatty acids
b) Glutamine
c) Glucose
d) Pyruvate

Primary fuel for Cancer cells and enterocytes is glutamine and for colonocytes, short chain fatty acids.

Stomach, Small Bowel, Spleen, Pancreas	Glutamine
Liver	Acetoacetate, Beta hydroxyl butyric acid: FFA
Neoplastic Cells	Glutamine
Prepheral nerves, adrenal medulla, RBC, PMN	Obligate glucose
Colon	Short chain FA (butyrate)

Answer B.

5) 65 year old male presents to the ER complaining of nausea, vomiting and obstipation for 2 days. Patient has previous history of cholecystectomy and appendectomy. CT scan of the Abd and pelvis showed sigmoid colon obstruction. Most likely diagnosis is:

a) Adhesions
b) Hernia
c) Volvulus
d) Neoplasia

SBO is more frequently caused by post-operative adhesions and hernias. Less frequently, tumors or strictures can cause intrinsic blockage. Most common cause of large bowel obstruction with or without previous surgery is cancer. Evaluation begins with plain x-rays of the abdomen and an upright CXR. CT scan has the resolution to assess the degree of obstruction and can also elucidate the cause. **Answer D.**

6) Which of the following is the most sensitive test for detecting Carcinoid tumor:

a) Urine 5-HIAA
b) Octreotide scan
c) Chromogranin A
d) Abdominal CT

In a report from the SEER database, the majority were located in the GI tract (55%) and bronchopulmonary system (30%). Within the GI tract, most carcinoids arose in the small intestine (45%, most commonly in the ileum), followed by rectum (20 %), appendix (16 %), colon (11%), and stomach (7%). Most common symptoms include diarrhea or flushing. The most useful initial diagnostic test for the carcinoid syndrome is to measure 24-hour urinary excretion of 5-HIAA. CT and Octreotide scan(more sensitive) are used for tumor localization. **Answer C.**

7) Which of the following is the most common site that presents with Carcinoid syndrome:

a) Colon
b) Ileum
c) Stomach
d) Appendix

45 % carcinoids appear in the Ileum followed by rectum (20%), appendix (16 %), colon (10%) and stomach (8%). **Answer B.**

8) 38 year old male with RLQ pain was found to have a 0.8 cm lesion at the mesoappendix. Intra operative frozen section reported Carcinoid tumor. Management includes:

a) Right hemicolectomy
b) Close the abdomen and Octreotide
c) Ileocecectomy with lymphnode dissection
d) Appendectomy only

Simple appendectomy is enough for tumors <2 cm that do not invade the mesoappendix. Right hemicolectomy is recommended for tumors >2 cm or with mesoappendiceal invasion. **Small bowel carcinoids** should undergo resection of the involved segment and mesentery. Pancreaticoduodenectomy has been advocated for resectable tumors at the ampulla. **Rectal carcinoids** that are smaller than 1 cm and confined to the mucosa or submucosa (T1) can be treated by local endoscopic excision. Tumors larger than 2 cm and those that invade into or beyond the muscularis propria or have regional lymph node metastases are treated by low anterior resection or APR. **Nonmetastatic colonic carcinoid** should be managed with partial colectomy and regional lymphadenectomy. For **type 1 and 2 gastric** carcinoids smaller than 1 cm, endoscopic resection is the treatment of choice. **Type 3** are treated by partial or total gastrectomy with local lymph node resection. **Answer A.**

9) 39 year old male, history of HIV, was admitted to the hospital with lower GI bleed. Work up confirmed small bowel lymphoma without metastasis. Treatment of choice is:

a) Radiotherapy followed by Chemotherapy
b) Chemotherapy only
c) Wide en block resection with negative margins only and lymphnode sampling
d) Triple antibiotic therapy

Lymphoma may involve the small intestine primarily or as a manifestation of disseminated systemic disease. Primary small intestinal lymphomas are most commonly located in the ileum, (highest concentration of lymphoid tissue in the intestine). 10% of patients with small intestinal lymphoma present with bowel perforation. Localized small intestinal lymphoma should be treated with **segmental resection** of the involved intestine and adjacent mesentery. If the small intestine is diffusely affected by lymphoma, chemotherapy rather than surgical resection should be the primary therapy. **The value to adjuvant chemotherapy after resection of localized lymphoma is controversial. Answer C.**

10) 60 year old male, presented to the ER with nausea, vomiting and obstipation for 6 hs, acute onset. CT scan showed intussusceptions at the ileocecal valve. Next step in management is:

a) Reduction with barium enema followed by bowel preparation and colonoscopy
b) Reduction with barium enema followed by resection
c) Colonoscopic detorsion followed by bowel preparation and resection
d) Resection

Adult intussusceptions are far less common, and usually have a distinct pathologic lead point, which can be malignant in up to one half of cases.They commonly present with a history of intermittent abdominal pain and signs and symptoms of bowel obstruction. CT scan is the investigation of choice, where a "target sign" may be seen. Treatment is **surgical resection** of the involved segment and the lead point, which needs to undergo pathologic evaluation to rule out an underlying malignancy. **Answer D.**

11) After resection of a long segment of small bowel, which of the following confirms the diagnosis of short bowel syndrome:

a) 60cm remnant with competent ileocecal valve
b) 100 cm remnant without ileocecal valve, off TPN
c) Sudan red stool stain and Schilling test
d) Inability to absorb enough water and nutrients

The most common etiologies of **short bowel syndrome** are acute mesenteric ischemia, malignancy, and Crohn's disease. Among adult patients who lack a functional colon, lifelong TPN dependence is likely to persist if there is less than **100 cm** of residual small intestine. Among adult patients who have an intact and functional colon, lifelong TPN dependence is likely to persist if there is less than **60 cm** of residual small intestine. Among infants with short bowel syndrome, weaning from TPN-dependence has been achieved with as little as 10 cm of residual small intestine. Diagnosis is based in symptoms, not in length, but in most cases, a) and b) are necessary to be off TPN. **Answer D.**

12) Which of the following recovers first from postoperative ileus:

a) Esophagus
b) Stomach
c) Small bowel
d) Colon

Postoperative ileus The small bowel generally recovers effective motor function within 24 hours after the operation; contractile activity in the small intestine remains present even during a celiotomy. In contrast, the stomach may take 24–48 hours to regain normal motor activity, while the colon recovers in about 3–5 days postoperatively.

Alvimopan, an oral peripherally acting mu-opioid receptor antagonist (PAM-OR) has limited ability to cross the blood brain barrier and is know to hasten post operative ileus in bowel surgery and abdominal hysterectomy. Alvimopan had a shown to reduce time to first passage of stool,early tolerance of regular diet, and reduced length of hospital stay in many randomized controlled trials. Many options suggested to reduce the postoperative ileus are:

- Gentle handling and minimal manipulation of the intestines
- Midthoracic epidurals with local anesthetics for postoperative pain control
- Minimally invasive surgery instead of laparotomy
- Limiting the length of laparotomy incisions
- Nonsteroidal antiinflammatory drugs instead of opioids for analgesia
- Delayed postoperative feeding, early ambulation, routine nasogastric tube placement, and pharmacologic therapy are not effective for preventing postoperative ileus.
Answer C.

13) Which of the following is the most common complication of Meckel's diverticulum in children:

a) Perforation
b) Bleeding
c) Inflammation
d) Obstruction

Meckel's diverticulum is the most prevalent congenital anomaly of the GI tract, 2% of the general population . Meckel's diverticula are true diverticula because their walls contain all of the layers found in normal small intestine. Their location varies and are usually found in the ileum within 100 cm of the ileocecal valve Bleeding associated with **Meckel's diverticulum** is usually the result of ileal mucosal ulceration that occurs adjacent to acid-producing, heterotopic gastric mucosa located within the diverticulum. The most common presentations are **bleeding**, intestinal obstruction, and diverticulitis. If the indication for diverticulectomy is bleeding (segmental resection of ileum that includes both the diverticulum and the adjacent ileal peptic ulcer should be performed), presence of a tumor or if the base of the diverticulum is inflamed or perforated. Radionuclide scans (^{99m}Tc-pertechnetate) may be helpful in the diagnosis of Meckel's diverticulum; if the diverticulum contains associated ectopic gastric mucosa that is capable of uptake of the tracer. In adults, the most common complication is **obstruction**.

Small bowel diverticula occur most frequently in the duodenum, however most are asymptomatic. Obstruction, food impaction, perforation, and bleeding are rare complications. These diverticula are also associated with a higher frequency of common bile duct stones due to external compression. The major clinical manifestation of **jejunoileal diverticula** is malabsorption due to bacterial overgrowth.

In asymptomatic patients with small bowel diverticula, observation is recommended. **Bacterial overgrowth** can be treated with antibiotics. Complications of jejunal diverticula including jejunoileal diverticulitis, bowel perforation, or bleeding, may require open or laparoscopic-assisted resection of the involved segment. **Answer B.**

14) Treatment of long segmentduodenal stricture from Crohn's disease include which of the following:

a) Whipple procedure
b) Stricturoplasty
c) Gastrojejunostomy with vagotomy
d) Segmental Duodenal resection.

Primary **Crohn's disease** of the duodenum almost always manifests with stricturing disease that can be managed by strictureplasty or with bypass procedures. When the duodenum is involved with Crohn's fistulas, it is always the result of disease within a distal segment (typically the terminal ileum or neo-terminal ileum) that fistulizes into an otherwise normal duodenum. Vagotomy is added to gastrojejunostomy since vagotomy protects jejunal mucosa from gastric acidity. **Answer C.**

15) A 75-year-old man has 30 lb weight loss for 3 months. Recently patient had noticed early satiety and vomiting. Computed tomographic (CT) scan demonstrates dialted stomach and 1st and 2nd portion of duodenum. Mass is noted in the 4th portion of the duodenum without involvement of SMA. The most appropriate management for this patient would be:

a) Pylorus preserving pancreaticoduodenectomy
b) Segmental duodenectomy with lymphadenectomy
c) Roux en Y Gastrojejunostomy
d) Chemoradiation

Whipple procedure is indicated in adenocarcinoma involving 2nd portion of duodenum, periampullary tumor. 3rd and 4th part of duodenum are treated like small bowel adenocarcinoma ie. Segmental resection with lymphadenectomy. **Answer B.**

16) Three years following an ileal resection, a 45 y/o male with short bowel syndrome has hematuria and flank pain. He passed several urinary small stones. Their composition is most likely:

a) Calcium oxalate
b) Calcium phosphate
c) Magnesium ammonium phosphate
d) Uric acid
e) Cysteine

There is increased absorption of **oxalate** following short

bowel syndrome or jejuno-ileal bypass in the colon as a result of increased delivery of soluble oxalate and possibly increased colonic permeability. In patient with terminal ileal resection, the mechanism of hyperoxaluria is through fat malabsorption and increased delivery of faecal fat to the colon. The fatty acids bind calcium to form soaps, leading to an increase in the concentration of the more soluble sodium oxalate absorbed in colon. Oxalate is excreted, precipitated to cause **Calcium oxalate** stones. As renal function declines, oxalate clearance also falls, causing higher plasma and tissue levels, which eventually cause accelerating tissue deposition of calcium oxalate. **Answer A**.

17) 71-year-old female that was treated for a stage III cancer of the cervix 8 years ago has chronic diarrhea and an acute small bowel obstruction. At operation, the serosa of the distal small intestine appears grey and opaque. This is characteristic of:

a) Crohns
b) Sprue
c) Niacin deficiency
d) Radiation

Radiation enteritis occurs usually 6 months following radiation therapy of various abdominal cancers. It affects small bowel and large bowel leading to diarrhea, nausea, constipation, bowel obstruction. Cervical cancer treatment may involve radiation with chemotherapy. If patient develops complete small bowel obstruction, surgery is warrented. During surgery diffuse fibrosis and adhesions between bowel loops makes dissection extremely tedious. Which increases the rate of leaks high due to poor blood supply to irradiated bowe. Extensive lysis of adhesion should be avoided as this exposis the patient to risk for enterocutaneous fistula and sepsis. Intestinal bypass is recommended to divert the proximal bowel from the site of obstruction. Also extensive resection may be neede due to severe adhesion, enterotomis and potentially leading to short bowel syndrome. **Answer D.**

18) The absorption of most dietary fat involves the formation of chylomicrons. These particules are:

a) Formed in the lumen of the small intestine
b) Manufactured in the enterocyte
c) The major route for cholesterol absorption
d) Rich in bile salts
e) Transported from the bowel by the portal venous system

Chylomicrons are lipoprotein particles synthesized in enterocytes for the transport of dietaty fat.
Triglycerides (85%), phospholipids (10%), cholesterol (2-3%) and proteins (1-2%) make up chylomicroms. The chylomicrons are transported through the thoracic duct as chyle. Chyle has a high content of triglycerides in the form of chylomicrons; Chyle also contains lymphocytes (primarily T lymphocytes) as the major cellular component and is bacteriostatic. Chyle is also rich in immunoglobulins and contains all of the fat soluble vitamins absorbed from the intestine. **Answer B.**

19) The major strength in an intestinal anastomosis is provided by the:

a) Lamina propria
b) Muscularis mucosa
c) Muscularis propria
d) Submucosa
e) Serosa

Submucosa is the strength layer of bowel which provides major strength of anastomosis. The Submucosa is the main layer responsible for holding the anastomosis and decreasing leak rate. As a result there is no difference in leakage rate between one layered vs two layer anastomsis. **Answer D.**

20) Vitamin K is mostly absorbed in which of the following part of the GI tract:

a) Stomach
b) Small bowel
c) Ascending Colon
d) Descending Colon

Antibiotics can cause **vitamin K deficiency** by decreasing **intestinal bacteria**, and also through direct effects on vitamin K activation in the liver. Most of the ingested vit K is absorbed in the distal small intestine. **Answer B.**

21) Proteins are mostly absorbed in which part of the GI tract:

a) Stomach
b) Jejunum
c) Ileum
d) Ascending Colon

Protein digestion begins in the **stomach** by the action of **pepsins**. In the **duodenum**, several **proteases** act together to digest proteins into AA, di or tripeptides. Malabsorption may occur when pancreatic protease secretion is impaired, as in chronic pancreatitis. **Answer B.**

22) Bile salts are mostly absorbed in which part of the gastrointestinal tract:

    a) Duodenum
    b) Jejunum
    c) Proximal ileum
    d) Distal ileum
    e) Ascending Colon

The **enterohepatic circulation** of bile salts occurs in the **distal ileum**. Fat **malabsorption** may occur when **resection of the terminal ileum** results in severe impairment of the enterohepatic circulation, and the liver's ability to increase bile acid synthesis is inadequate to meet physiological needs for bile production. **Answer D**.

23) Which of the following substances are absorbed in the jejunum:

    a) Water, sodium, fat and folic acid
    b) Water, potassium, carbohydrates with Vitamin B12
    c) Water, sodium, proteins and bile acids
    d) Water, carbohydrates and bile acids

Bile acids are reabsorbed in **terminal ileum**- enterohepatic circulation. **Vit B12** binds to intrinsic factor in the stomach and is reabsorbed in the **terminal ileum**. **Answer A.**

17. COLON, RECTUM AND ANUS

1) Regarding blood supply to the rectum, the Middle rectal artery is a branch of:

   a) Internal Pudendal Artery
   b) Left Colic Artery
   c) Internal Iliac Artery
   d) External Iliac Artery

   SMA branches include the Ileocolic, Right colic and middle colic arteries. IMA branches are the Left colic, sigmoidal and Superior rectal arteries. The superior rectal artery is the continuation of the inferior mesenteric artery. It descends into the pelvis between the layers of the mesentery of the sigmoid colon, crossing the left common iliac artery and vein. Middle rectal artery arises from internal iliac artery and runs in the lateral rectal ligaments. Internal pudendal artery is a branch of the Internal iliac and supplies the lower rectum. **Answer C.**

2) Regarding the watershed areas in the colorectal circulation, which of the following is true:

   a) Griffith's point (splenic flexure) is formed by the Middle Colic and right colic arteries
   b) Griffith's point is formed by the Left colic and sigmoidal arteries junction
   c) Sudeck's point in the rectum is formed by the superior and middle rectal arteries
   d) Sudeck's point is formed by the Middle and inferior rectal arteries junction

Arterial **supply** to the colon comes from branches of the superior mesenteric artery (SMA) and inferior mesenteric artery (IMA). Flow between these two systems communicates via a "marginal artery" that runs parallel to the colon for its entire length. Watershed points are areas of poor collateral circulation in the colon, more susceptible to ischemia. **Griffith's point** is formed by the IMA and SMA junction. **Sudeck's point** is formed by Superior rectal and Middle rectal junction. 80% of blood flow goes to mucosa and submucosa. **Answer C**.

3) 63 year old male, complaining of weight loss and cough was found to have a lung mass in CXR. CT guided biopsied confirmed the lesion to be metastatic from the rectum. Which of the following pathway for this metastasis is true:

a) Inferior rectal vein draining into the Internal iliac vein then IVC
b) Middle Rectal vein draining into the Internal Iliac vein then IVC
c) Superior Rectal vein draining into the IMV
d) Internal pudendal artery draining into the IMV

Patients can get lung metastasis from low rectal cancer because the inferior rectal vein drains into the Internal iliac and eventually into the IVC, reaching the lungs. Whereas Ascending, Transverse, Descending, Sigmoid colon and Superior rectal cancer typically metastatize to liver as SMV, IMV drain into portal vein. **Answer A**.

4) Regarding defecation control and anal sphincter anatomy, which of the following is true:

a) Internal anal sphincter is a continuation of the puborectalis muscle
b) Internal sphincter control does not depend on the pudendal nerves integrity
c) External sphincter is innervated by the pelvic splanchnic nerves
d) External anal sphincter is a continuation of the muscularis propria

External anal sphincter (voluntary control) is a continuation of the puborectalis muscle and under CNS control (Pudendal nerves-sympathetic). Internal sphincter (involuntary control) is the continuation of the muscularis propria and innervated by pelvic splanchnic branches (Parasympathetic). **Answer B.**

5) Which of the following is the main nutrient for colonocytes:

a) Glutamine
b) Short chain fatty acids
c) Pyruvate
d) Alanine

Short chain fatty acids (SCFAs) are the products of colonic bacterial degradation of unabsorbed starch and non-starch Polysaccharide (fibre). They are important anions in the colonic lumen, affecting both colonocyte morphology and function. The three main acids (**acetate, propionate, and butyrate**) stimulate colonic sodium and fluid absorption and exert proliferative effects on the colonocyte. Glutamine is the main source for enterocytes and cancer cells. **Answer B.**

6) 65 year old male presented to your office 4 weeks after total abdominal colectomy and ileostomy for perforated diverticulitis. Patient is complaining of mild fever and purulent drainage from the rectum. Colonoscopy showed inflammation and friable mucosa. Correct management is:

a) Short chain fatty acid enemas
b) Steroid enemas
c) Cipro and Flagyl
d) Low anterior resection

Short chain fatty acids should be used to treat disuse pouchitis (Hartman's) .Treatment of infectious pouchitis is metronidazole (Flagyl). Treatment of Lymphocytic colitis (watery diarrhea and inflammatory bowel symptoms) is sulfasalazine. **Answer C**.

7) Regarding Ulcerative colitis all of the following are true , except:

a) Surgery is not curative
b) Spares anus
c) Total colectomy is indicated if any dysplasia is found on colonoscopy
d) Steroid is the best medical treatment for acute exacerbations

UC usually presents with bloody diarrhea, abdominal pain, fever, weight loss. It involves mucosa and submucosa (transmural in Crohn's) Strictures and fistulae unusual with ulcerative colitis. Spares anus -unlike Crohn's diease. It starts distally in rectum, is contiguous (no skip areas like Crohn's disease) Bleeding is universal and has mucosal friability with pseudopolyps and collar button ulcers. Diagnosis with Colonoscopy with biopsy. Treament is with.
1) Sulfasalazine + 5-ASA- mild disease.
2) Steroids - to induce remission.
3) Methotrexate, azathioprine: moderate to severe flare up.
4) Infliximab - monoclonal antibody against TNF-alpha. 5-ASA and sulfasalazine have been shown to maintain remission in ulcerative colitis. Surgical indications include failed medical therapy, worsening toxic megacolon, any dysplasia, Cancer, significant hemorrhage, perforation and failure to thrive. **Answer A.**

8) After total abdominal colectomy for Ulcerative colitis, which of the following does **not** improve:

   a) Anemia
   b) Ankylosing Spondylitis
   c) Arthritis
   d) Ocular

   Primary Sclerosing cholangitis and Ankylosing Spondylitis (HLA-B27) does not improve and Pyoderma gangrenosum improves in 50% of the patients. Anemia, Arthritis, Ocular symptoms improve with Total abdominal colectomy.
   Answer B.

9) 49 year old male, history of Crohn's disease controlled with 5-ASA drug, now presents to your clinic complaining of new onset drainage from his abdominal wall since last week. On physical exam you notice small amount of enteric contents drainage but no cellulitis or pus. The following drug should be added to this patient regimen:

a) Prednisone
b) Loperamide
c) Infliximab
d) Methotrexate

In patients with Crohn's disease, Infliximab and Flagyl have been shown to be effective in healing fistulas (enterocutaneous, colovesical) Infliximab can cause TB reactivation. Surgical resection is not known to cause remission of Crohn's disease unlike UC. Medical treatment is same as UC (refer to question -8). However surgical options include stricturoplasty, Total abdominal colectomy with end ileostomy. **Answer C.**

10) Which of the following operative finding is not common in patients with Crohn's disease:

a) Cobblestoning in the rectum
b) Skip lesion in the sigmoid
c) Creeping mesenteric fat
d) Transmural involvement

Unlike UC, Crohn's disease usually spares the rectal, affects the anus (fissures→ no sphincterotomy indicated), fistulas are present and involvement is segmental. **Fat wrapping** is the most commonly seen during exploratory laparotomy. Treatment of Crohn's fistula includes resection of involved segment with primary anastomosis. However involvement of Duodenum mandates either stricturoplasty vs Gastrojejunostomy. (Whipple is not indicated). **Answer A.**

11) All of the following are complications from terminal ileum resection, **except**:

a) Gallstones formation because of decreased bile salt uptake
b) Megaloblastic anemia because of decreased vitamin B12 uptake
c) Kidney stones because of increased Calcium-oxalate binding
d) Diarrhea because of decreased bile salt uptake

Because of decreased calcium-oxalate binding, oxalate is absorbed and patient develops hyperoxaluria. **Answer C.**

12) 72 year old female brought to the ER from nursing home with history of chronic constipation, arthritis (on narcotics), and abdominal distention for the past 5 days. Patient is afebrile and hemodinamically stable. Physical exam evidenced significant abdominal distention but no peritoneal signs. CT scan showed large bowel dilation without masses with Cecum measuring 14 cm. Management includes all of the following, **except**:

a) NGT placement and electrolytes replacement
b) Neostigmine 2.5mg IV
c) Colonoscopy
d) Cecostomy

Major cause of Colonic obstruction includes Cancer (#1 cause), Volvulus, Diverticulitis, and IBD. **Diagnosis** of Ogilvie's SD (Psuedoobstruction) – AXR massive diffuse dilated colon. It is treated with NGT, NPO, and IVF hydration. Potassium K^+ level > 4. Neostigmine 2.5 mg IV should be given if above fails (Keep atropine handy for Bradycardia associated with Neostigmine) . Colonoscopic decompression should be attempted if cecum is larger than 12cm or failure of medical treatment 24-48 hr. If colonoscopy fails or free air is noted, cecostomy or right hemicolectomy w/ colostomy and mucus fistula can be performed. **Answer D.**

13) 63 year old male, history of chronic constipation, presented to the ER complaining of acute onset RLQ pain associated with nausea and vomiting. Patient was afebrile, hemodinamically stable and without peritoneal signs. CT scan showed closed loop obstruction, small bowel obstruction and dilated cecum. Correct management is:

   a) Bowel rest, NGT placement, correct electrolytes and observation in ICU
   b) Barium enema
   c) Right colectomy with primary anastomosis
   d) Colonoscopic decompression, bowel preparation and colectomy in same admission

Cecum Volvulus is very hard to detorse, so barium enema or colonoscopy should not be attempted as in cases of sigmoid volvulus. AXR reveals Ace of Spade appearance. Right hemicolectomy with primary anastomosis is the best treatment. Cecopexy has higher failure rates. **Answer C.**

14) 41 year old female, history of chronic constipation, presented to the ER complaining of fever, nausea and left lower quadrant pain for the past 48 hs. WBC was 18.000 and CT scan showed inflammation around the sigmoid colon with 3cm pelvic abscess. Correct management is:

a) Bowel rest, IV fluids, IV antibiotics and ICU admission
b) Colonoscopy
c) IV antibiotics and Percutaneous drainage
d) Hartman's procedure

Hinchey classification of Diverticulitis
- Stage I — pericolic or mesenteric abscess
- Stage II — walled-off pelvic abscess
- Stage III — generalized purulent peritonitis
- Stage IV — generalized fecal peritonitis

Uncomplicated diverticulitis (Hinchey I, II) should be managed conservatively with NPO/IV antibiotics. Complicated diverticulitis with abscess (Hinchey III) should be treated with percutaneous drainage and, if perforation or fecal peritonitis is present (Hinchey IV), surgery is indicated.
Answer C.

15) Which of the following gene mutation is not typically associated with colorectal cancer:

a) K-ras
b) p-53
c) DCC
d) RET

APC and p-53 (tumor suppressor genes), K-ras (oncogene) and DCC are the main gene mutations involved in colorectal cancer. hMSH2, hMLH1, hPMS1 and hPMS2 are DNA mismatch genes associated with Lynch Syndrome.
Answer D.

16) Which of the following adenomas does not have increased risk of colon cancer:

a) Hyperplastic
b) >2cm
c) Villous
d) Sessile

Tubular adenomas have **5** % risk of developing colon cancer, Tubulo-villous 20% and Villous **40%** chance. Increased cancer risk features include **> 2 cm, villous, sessile lesions. Answer A**.

17) Which of the following is the most important prognostic factor in colorectal cancer:

a) CEA level
b) Mitotic rate
c) Tumor grade
d) Lymphnode status

CEA is not useful for screening, but may suggest recurrence. Colon cancer usually spreads first to lymphnodes. Various porgnostic factors per consensus of American Pathologist are: the local **extent of tumor** assessed pathologically (T), regional **lymph node** metastasis (the pN category of the TNM staging system**); blood or lymphatic vessel invasion**; residual tumor following surgery with curative intent ,especially as it relates to **positive surgical margins;** and preoperative elevation of **carcinoembryonic antigen elevation** (CEA). **Answer D**.

18) In colon cancer, a T2 lesion is defined by:

a) Involves mucosa only
b) Penetrates through muscularis mucosa and into submucosa
c) Penetrates through submucosa and into muscularis propria
d) Penetrates through muscularis propria and into subserosal

Option A is Tis, B is T1 and option D describes a T3 lesion. T4 lesion penetrates through serosa or involves adjacent organs. Involvement of **Lymph nodes** makes the lesion Stage III. Metastasis to distant organs is StageIV.**Answer C.**

19) Standard colon resection is based in which anatomic structure:

a) Lymphnode drainage
b) Venous drainage
c) Arterial supply
d) Retroperitoneal attachments

For a right hemicolectomy, the Ileocolic and right colic should be divided; Transverse colectomy involves division of the middle colic and left hemicolectomy involves division of the left colic artery. For right or left extended colectomies, the middle colic should be divided. **Subtotal colectomy**: entire colon except sigmoid and rectum are revomce. **Total colectomy**: entire colon, sigmoid colon in removed except rectum.**Total proctocolectomy**: the entire colon, rectum, and anus are removed and the ileum is brought to the skin as a Brooke ileostomy. **Answer C.**

20) 70 year old male with low rectal tumor biopsy showing T1 lesion. Transanal excision is indicated, **except**:

a) If only 2mm margin can be obtained
b) Involves less than 1/3 of circumference
c) No neurovascular invasion
d) Tumor is less then 6cm

Criteria for Transanal Excision
- Less than 4 cm
- Location 8cm or less from anal verge
- Well or moderately differentiated histology
- Mobile, non ulcerated mass
- No suspicion of perirectal or presacral nodes
- Tumor involves less than 1/3 of circumference of the rectal wall
- Tumor stage T1 (mucosa and submucosa)
Answer D.

21) 61 year old male with history of sigmoid cancer now presents with liver metastasis. Poor prognostic factors include all of the following , **except**:

a) Size more than 5cm
b) More than 3 lesions
c) CEA level greater than 50 ug/L
d) Synchronous primary cancer

Poor prognostic factors in patients with liver metastasis:
- Disease free interval < 12 months,
- > 3 Tumors,
- CEA > 200(ug/L),
- Size > 5 cm,
- Positive nodes,
- Synchronous primary and liver mets.
Answer C.

22) 52 year old male presents to the ER complaining of severe weakness & dizziness. Work up reveals severe anemia and occult bleeding on fecal blood testing. Next step in management is:

a) Anoscopy
b) Proctoscopy
c) EGD
d) Colonoscopy

Occult bleeding refers to the initial presentation of a positive fecal occult blood test (FOBT) and/or iron deficiency anemia when there is no evidence of visible blood loss to the patient or physician. Patients with a positive FOBT and anemia should be evaluated with upper **endoscopy and colonoscopy**. If these studies are unrevealing, small bowel source of bleeding should be ruled out preferably with capsule endoscopy. **Answer C.**

23) Which of the following describes Tertiary internal hemorrhoids:

a) Prolapse slides below dentate line with strain
b) Prolapse reduces spontaneously
c) Prolapse must be reduced manually
d) Prolapse does not reduce

Internal hemorrhoids are classified as:

Grade I: The hemorrhoids do not prolapse. **Grade II:** The hemorrhoids prolapse upon valsalva and reduce spontaneously **Grade III:** The hemorrhoids prolapse and must be reduced manually **Grade IV:** The hemorrhoids are prolapsed and cannot be reduced manually.

Rx Dietary management consisting of adequate fluid and fiber intake as the primary medical treatment of symptomatic hemorrhoids. For medically refractory **grades I and II** hemorrhoids, rubber band ligation as the initial office-based procedure. For patients with a **single** symptomatic grade **III** hemorrhoid, the authors perform a rubber band ligation. If **two or three** hemorrhoidal columns are symptomatic: surgical excision. For patients with grade **IV** hemorrhoids or who have combined internal and external hemorrhoids with significant prolapsed: surgical excision. **Answer C.**

24) 74 year old female presented with hematochezia for the past 2 weeks. Endoscopic USG with biopsy showed a 4cm Squamous cell carcinoma 1cm **below** the dentate line and negative lymphnodes. Correct management is:

a) Chemoradiation therapy
b) Radiation followed by transanal excision
c) Wide local excision
d) Abdominoperineal resection

Wide local excision with 1cm margin can be performed for tumors located below the dentate line (Anal margin lesions), less then 5cm in size and with negative nodes. **Answer C.**

25) Which colonic bacteria is the most common:

a) Escherichia coli
b) Klebsiella
c) Bacteroides
d) Enterococcus

Approximately 90% of the dry weight of feces is composed of bacteria, of which **Bacteroides vulgatus** is the most common. **Answer C**.

26) What is the most common genetic syndrome associated with colorectal cancer:

a) HNPCC
b) FAP
c) Juvenile Polyposis
d) Crohn's disease

Approximately 5% of colorectal carcinomas are associated with genetic syndromes of which HNPCC is the most common. The lifetime risk of developing colon cancer in Lynch syndrome is approximately 70 percent (100% in FAP). Amsterdam II criteria **3-2-1 rule** (3 affected members, 2 generations, 1 under age 50). **Answer A.**

27) Which of these statements regarding Hirschsprung's Disease is false:

a) Occurs in children and adults
b) Absence of ganglion cells
c) More common in males
d) Unopposed parasympathetic tone

Hirschsprung's disease is caused by the failure of the parasympathetic myenteric nerve cells to migrate to the distal colon. Unopposed sympathetic tone causes a functional obstruction. **Rectal biopsy** is considered the gold standard for diagnosis. The treatment is surgical resection of the aganglionic segment of bowel. The normal ganglionic bowel is brought down and anastomosed to the anus, and sphincter function is generally preserved (Laparoscopic assisted and transanal repairs). **Answer D.**

28) The colonic mucosa crypts are lined by all of these cells, **except**:

   a) Goblet cells
   b) APUD cells
   c) Enterochromaffin cells
   d) Parietal cells

   Parietal cells secret HCl and are found in the gastric mucosa. **Answer D.**

29) Meissner's plexus is located in which layer of the colon:

   a) Mucosa
   b) Submucosa
   c) Muscularis propria
   d) Adventitia

   The submucosa contains the vessels, lymphatics and Meissner's plexus (parasympathetic plexus) Auerbach's plexus exists between the longitudinal and circular layers of muscularis externa in the gastrointestinal tract. (MeIssNNER - Inner submucosa. Auerbach: a**OUTER**bach muscularis externa). **Answer B.**

30) Complications associated with ulcerative colitis includes:

   a) Intestinal obstruction
   b) Cholelithiasis
   c) Nephrolithiasis
   d) Sclerosing cholangitis

Intestinal obstruction, cholelithiasis, and nephrolithiasis are associated with Crohn's disease.

Endoscopic findings include: Loss of the vascular appearance of the colon Erythema (or redness of the mucosa) and friability of the mucosa, Superficial **ulceration**, which may be confluent, and **Pseudopolyp**. There is a significantly **increased risk** of colorectal cancer in patients with ulcerative colitis after ten years if involvement is beyond the splenic flexure. Those with only proctitis or rectosigmoiditis usually have no increased risk. **Pancolitis and younger age** have increased association with colon cancer. It is recommended that patients have screening colonoscopies with random biopsies to look for dysplasia after eight years of disease activity. Extraintestinal manifestations are uveitis, Primary sclrosing cholangitis, Ankylosing spondylitis, pyoderma gangrenosum and Erythema Nodosum. **Answer D.**

31) Which of these is **false** regarding Clostridium Difficile Colitis:

a) C. difficile is a gram +, anaerobic organism
b) Clindamycin is the primary culprit
c) Antidiarrheal agents should be avoided
d) Pseudomembranous colitis

Any antibiotic can potentially cause C. diff colitis and initial treatment is cessation of it. Metronidazole is indicated for non-severe forms of C. Diff colitis. Vancomycin PO is used for the treatment of severe disease. Surgical evaluation should be considered for patients ≥65 years with WBC ≥20,000 and/or lactate level between 2.2 and 4.9 meq/L. Subtotal colectomy with end ileostomy is the procedure of choice in the setting of peritoneal signs, severe ileus, or toxic megacolon. **Answer B.**

32) What are the sites for colonic volvulus in decreasing order:

a) Sigmoid, Right colon, Transverse
b) Sigmoid, Transverse, Right colon
c) Right colon, Sigmoid, Transverse
d) Transverse, Sigmoid, Right colon

61% occur in the sigmoid colon. **Answer A**.

33) A mutation in the p53 gene plays a major role in the development of colorectal cancer. What is the definition of p53 gene:

a) Oncogene
b) Mismatch repair gene
c) VEGF
d) Tumor suppressor

p53 (chromosome **17**) is a tumor suppressor gene that inhibits cellular proliferation. In about 50 to 70 percent of colorectal ca, p53 inactivation occurs. APC tumor suppressor gene (chromosome **5**) mutations are present in 80 percent of sporadic CRCs, and a single germline mutation in this gene is responsible for FAP. **Answer D.**

34) Carcinoembryonic antigen can be elevated in a variety of cancers including:

a) Colorectal
b) Bone
c) Ovarian
d) Pancreatic

CEA is a useful marker for a variety of cancers. Carcinoembryonic antigen (CEA) is a glycoprotein involved in cell adhesion. It is elevated in serum from individuals with colorectal carcinoma, gastric carcinoma, pancreatic carcinoma, lung carcinoma and breast carcinoma, as well as individuals with medullary thyroid carcinoma, had higher levels of CEA than healthy individuals (above 2.5 ng/ml). CEA measurement is mainly used as a tumor marker to identify **recurrences** after surgical resection. The CEA blood test is **not** reliable for diagnosing cancer or as a screening test for early detection of cancer. Most types of cancer do not produce a high CEA. Elevated CEA levels should return to normal after successful surgical resection or within 6 weeks of starting treatment if cancer treatment is successful. **Answer A.**

35) Which of the following is the procedure of choice in a 80 year old female with co morbidities presenting with rectal prolapse:

a) Levatorplasty
b) Perineal rectosigmoidectomy
c) Sacralpexy with sigmoidectomy
d) Posterior colporrhaphy

Grades of Rectal Prolapse. **First degree prolapse** is detectable below the anorectal ring on straining. **Second degree** when it reached the dentate line. **Third degree** when it reached the anal verge. Operations can be categorized as either *abdominal* or *perineal*. **Pt with Good condition** Transabdominal proctopexy for rectal prolapsed: The fully mobilized rectum is sutured to the presacral fascia. If desired, a sigmoid colectomy can be performed concomitantly to resect the redundant colon. **Old frail patient:** Perineal rectosigmoidectomy: A circular incision is made 2 cm proximal to the dentate line. The redundant bowel is resected. A handsewn anastomosis is performed between sigmoid/rectum to anus. It is associated with less morbidity but has higher recurrence. **Answer B.**

36) 63 year old male was found to have 6 adenomatous polyp in his screening colonoscopy. Patient denies family history of colon cancer or other malignancies. When does colonoscopic surveillance should be performed:

a) 2-6 months
b) 1 year
c) 3 year
d) 5 years

According to the most recent Guideline for Post polypectomy Surveillance for early detection of Colorectal Cancer , patients with small **hyperplastic polyps** should have colonsocpy in **10** yr. Patients with **1-2** small tubular adenomas should repeat colonoscopy in **5-10** years after polypectomy; Patients with **3-10** adenomas should repeat colonoscopy in **3** years; Patients with **> 10** adenomas should repeat in **< 3** years and patients with **sessile adenomas** removed piecemeal , should have a repeat colonoscopy in **2-6** months. **Answer C**.

37) How many layers are seen on Endoscopic Rectal Ultrasound:

a) 3
b) 4
c) 5
d) 7

The innermost layer (lumen) is known as the superficial mucosal layer. The 2nd layer corresponds to the lamina propria, the 3rd is the submucosa, the 4th is the muscularis propria, and the 5th is the **adventitia** in the esophagus and **serosa** in the rest of the GI tract. **Answer C.**

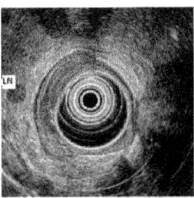

38) 83 year old female who has history of sever dementia now presented with abdominal distension for the past 2 weeks. AXR shows dilated large bowel with tapering in left lower quadrant. Correct management is:

a) Sigmodeopexy
b) Hartman's procedure
c) Sigmoidectomy
d) Loop colostomy

The majority of patients with sigmoid volvulus present with abdominal pain, nausea, abdominal distension, and constipation; vomiting is less common. However, some patients (particularly younger patients) may have a more insidious presentation with recurrent attacks of abdominal pain, with resolution presumably due to spontaneous detorsion. **Answer C.**

39) A 75 -year-old man undergoes low anterior resection of a rectal adenocarcinoma 7 cm from the anal verge. Final pathology reveals T2 lesion with 5 nodes positive. Which of the following statement is appropriate for postoperative adjuvant therapy:

a) Radiation therapy to the pelvis
b) Radiation therapy to the pelvis, para-aortic lymph nodes
c) Chemotherapy with 5 FU and levamisoel
d) Chemotherapy (FOLFOX) with radiaton to pelvic nodes.

Postoperative combined modality therapy over surgery alone is preferred for patients with resected stage II and III rectal cancer. Use of FOLFOX in this setting for a total of four to six months is recommended. FOLFOX is based upon an extrapolation of data from adjuvant treatment of colon cancer, and there is no evidence that FOLFOX is better that fluoropyrimidine therapy alone in the adjuvant setting of rectal cancer. **Answer D**.

40) 40 year old man is S/P proctocolectomy with ileoanal anastomosis for FAP. Recently patient has been complaining of increasing abdominal distension, abdominal pain relieved by a large bowel movements. A CT scan obtained is shown below.

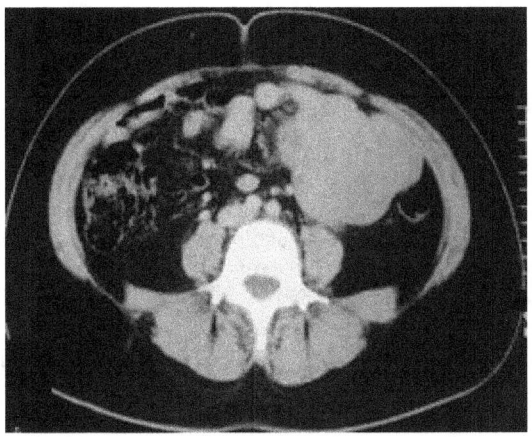

Which of the following is true about this condition:

a) Conservative management with tamoxifen or NSAID is optimal
b) Wide resection with negative margin
c) After resection, low recurrence is noted.
d) Pt treated with FAP, desmoids tumors are least cause of death.

Desmoid tumors are benign, slow growing neoplasms with no metastatic potential but a high risk for local recurrence. They are locally infiltrative and can cause death through destruction of adjacent vital structures. The risk is increased in patients with FAP (Gardner's syndrome). Observation is advocatedy for stable, asymptomatic desmoids. Surgical excision is indicated in symptomatic patients. Radiation therapy is an option for patients who are not good surgical candidates. **Answer B.**

41) 71 year old male presented to the ER complaining of nausea, fever and RLQ pain for the past 5 days. CT scan showed phlegmon around a walled off appendix. Next step in management is:

a) NPO and IV antibiotics
b) NPO and percutaneous drainage
c) Laparoscopic appendectomy
d) Colonoscopy to rule out perforated cancer

Treatment options for appendiceal phlegmon include immediate appendectomy or percutaneous drainage, typically with interval appendectomy. Patients who develop an appendiceal abscess respond best to initial **percutaneous drainage** and IV antibiotics. This may avoid the potential need for extended bowel resection.
Recent sstudies demonstrated that interval appendectomy is controversial because of the low recurrence rate.
Colonoscopy or barium enema should be performed to rule out colonic disease as the etiology before surgical intervention. **Answer A.**

42) 42 year old male presented to the ER complaining of anorexia and RLQ pain for the past 24hs. CT scan showed mild inflammatory changes around the appendix. Intra operative, the base of the appendix was uninvolved by terminal ileitis. Next step is:

a) Right hemicolectomy
b) Appendectomy
c) Intraoperative colonoscopy
d) Close the abdomen

Appendectomy should be performed if intraoperative, regional terminal ileitis is found and not involving the cecum. If it happens again, it will be one less differential diagnosis. **Answer B.**

18. HERNIAS

1) Medial boundary of the femoral canal is:

   a) Inguinal ligament
   b) Lacunar ligament
   c) Femoral vein
   d) Iliacus & psoas tendons and fascia of pectineus

   Femoral triangle is bounded by following:
   Superior- inguinal ligament
   Medial - lacunar ligament
   Lateral - femoral vein
   Posterior (floor)- iliacus & psoas tendons and fascia of pectineus
   Femoral hernias account for 2 to 4 percent of groin hernias, are more common in women, and are more apt to present with strangulation and require emergency surgery.
   Answer B.

2) Which of the following structure forms the inguinal ligament::

   a) Fascia transversalis
   b) External oblique fascia
   c) Internal oblique fascia
   d) Pectineal ligaments

   External oblique also forms the anterior aspect of the inguinal canal and the shelving edge (inferior portion). Internal oblique fascia joins with the transversalis fascia and forms the conjoint tendon. For treatment of Inguinal hernia strategy of **watchful waiting** rather than referral for surgery can be considered in patients with asymptomatic or minimally symptomatic inguinal hernia, as long as they are aware of the risk, albeit small, of hernia complications and understand the need for prompt medical attention should symptoms of these complications occur. **Answer B.**

263

3) Pectineal ligament is localized:

a) Superior to the femoral vessels
b) Inferior to the femoral vessels
c) Anterior to the femoral vessels
d) Posterior to the femoral vessels

Also known as cooper ligament, the pectineal ligament is posterior to the femoral vessels. Used in McVay repair to correct femoral hernias. It is an extension of the lacunar ligamentthat runs on the pectineal line of the pubic bone. The **inguinal ligament** is a band running from the pubic tubercle to the anterior superior iliac spine. **Answer D.**

4) Regarding inguinal hernia classification, which of the following is true:

a) Direct hernias are caused by weakness of the abdominal wall and located superior and medial to epigastric vessels
b) Indirect hernias are the most common type , located inferior and lateral to the epigastric vessels and are caused by patent processus vaginalis
c) Pantaloon hernias have direct and indirect components
d) Most common organ involved in sliding hernias is the bladder

Direct hernias are inferior and medial, Indirect hernias are superior and lateral, sliding hernias more commonly involve the sigmoid or cecum in males, and in females, the ovaries. A pantaloon hernia occurs when both a direct and an indirect hernia develop on the same side. Amyand's hernia: contains the appendix; Petit's hernia passes through inferior lumbar triangle, and Grynfeltt's hernia passes through superior lumbar triangle.
Answer C.

5) Regarding inguinal hernia repair, the Bassini technique consists of the approximation of:

a) Conjoint tendon to the pectineal ligament
b) Transversalis fascia to the conjoint tendon
c) Conjoint tendon and transversalis fascia to the shelving edge
d) Lacunar ligament to the shelving edge

Option A describes McVay repair for femoral hernia. Lichtenstein repair consist of mesh placement between the conjoint tendon and inguinal ligament (less recurrence). **Bassini repair** is non mesh repair where the weakened inguinal floor is strengthened by approximating the conjoined tendon to the inguinal ligament from the pubic tubercle medially to the area of the internal ring laterally. **Answer C.**

6) Which of the following is the most common early complication following inguinal hernia repair:

a) Ischemic orchitis
b) Medial thigh paresthesia
c) Urinary retention
d) Constipation

Answer C. Ischemic orchitis occurs in less than 1%, caused by thrombosis of the spermatic cord veins.

7) Which of the following nerve is most commonly injured during inguinal hernia repair:

a) Genital branch of the Genitofemoral Nerve
b) Femoral branch of the Genitofemoral Nerve
c) Pudendal Nerve
d) Ilioinguinal Nerve

The **genital branch of the genitofemoral** supplies the **cremaster** muscle the scrotal skin, and labia majora. The *femoral branch* supplies the skin anterior to the upper part of the femoral triangle. **Ilioinguinal nerve** suppplies the skin of the upper and medial part of the thigh, and is the most common injured nerveduring inguinal repair. Genitofemoral Nerve is the most commonly injured nerve during laparoscopic repair**Answer D.**

8) Which of the following is the most common cause of recurrence after Laparoscopic inguinal hernia repair:

a) Lateral separation of the mesh
b) Medial separation of the mesh
c) Superior separation of the mesh
d) Inferior separation of the mesh

Medial separation of the mesh from the fascia at the inguinal ligament. **Answer B**.

9) 81 year old female presented to the ER complaining of nausea and vomiting for the past 2 days. Patient is emaciated with abdominal distension. Flat and Upright X-ray showed air fluid levels below and above the pubic ramus. Correct management is:

a) Bowel rest , NGT placement and observation in the ICU
b) Bowel rest , NGT placement and Neostigmine 2,5mg IV
c) Bowel rest, NGT placement and colonoscopic decompression
d) Bowel rest, NGT placement and Operative reduction

An **obturator hernia** is caused by abdominal content protruding through the obturator foramen. Diagnosis is often made intraoperatively after presenting with bowel obstruction. The Howship-Romberg sign is suggestive and characterized by excruciating pain in the medial thigh, caused by compression of the obturator nerve. All obturator hernias require surgery to reduce the hernia and assess bowel viability. **Answer D.**

10) 2 year old African American male was noted to have a 2cm umbilical hernia on routine physical exam. Regarding this condition, which of the following is true:

a) Repair should be delayed until age 5
b) Hernias larger then 1.5cm in diameter should be repaired
c) High risk of incarceration in children
d) Repair should be performed with mesh

Most umbilical hernias < 2.5cm reduce spontaneously before age 5 and they rarely incarcerate. **Answer A.**

11) What is the definition of a Richter's hernia:

a) A hernia with the antimesenteric wall of intestine
b) Combined indirect and direct hernia
c) Femoral hernia
d) Lumbar hernia

A **Richter's** hernia is an abdominal hernia in which only **part of the circumference of the bowel** is entrapped in the defect. Symptoms are usually of a **partial SBO**, and may have local inflammation. The most common site is in the femoral canal followed by laparoscopic port sites. A **Spigelian** hernia occurs along the semilunar line because of the absence of a posterior sheath behind the rectus muscle. They have a high rate of incarceration and operative repair is recommended. **Answer A.**

12) Which layer of the abdominal wall gives rise to the Poupart's ligament:

a) Transverse
b) Internal oblique
c) External oblique
d) Lacunar ligament

External oblique fascia forms the inguinal ligament-Shelving edge-poupart ligament. Forms the anterior portion of inguinal canal. Internal oblique: muscle portion makes the cremasteric muscles. Fascia portion combines with transversalis fascia to form the conjoined tendon which serves the floor of the inguinal canal. Lacunar ligament connects the inguinal and pectineal ligament. Femoral vessels and nerve passes through that arc. External ring: entrance to canal from peritoneum. Hesselbach's triangle: rectus muscle, inferior inguinal ligament, inferior epigastric. Direct hernia is medial and inferior to the epigastric vessels, less likely to be strangulated, and indirect hernias are more common. **Answer C.**

13) All of the following form the boundaries of the femoral canal, **except**:

a) Iliopubic tract
b) Cooper's ligament
c) Femoral Vein
d) Femoral artery

Femoral hernias account for <10% of all groin hernias, but 40% present with incarceration or strangulation .The reason for the higher incidence in women may relate to the less bulky musculature, or weakness of the pelvic floor from childbirth. **Elective femoral hernias** should be approached with an infrainguinal incision and a small plug placed into the defect. The plug can be sutured to the inguinal ligament superiorly and the Cooper ligament medially. **Answer D.**

14) All of the following nerves are at risk for injury during an inguinal hernia repair, **except**:

a) Iliohypogastric
b) Pudendal
c) Genitofemoral
d) Ilioinguinal

Illioinguinal nerve injury results in loss of cremastric reflex, numbness of ipsilateral scrotum and inner thigh. Lateral femoral cutaneous and GFNare more likely to be injured during laparoscopic repair. The **genital branch** supplies the **cremaster** muscle the scrotal skin, and labia majora. The **femoral branch** supplies the skin anterior to the upper part of the femoral triangle. **Answer B.**

15) Most umbilical hernias close spontaneously at what age:

a) 2 years
b) 6 months
c) 12 years
d) Never

Most umbilical hernias close by age 2, persistent hernias after the age of 5 should be repaired primarily . In adults with defects that are 1 to 3cm, regardless of the method and mesh chosen, the placement of the product behind the musculature of the abdominal wall will provide the most durable repair . **Answer A.**

16) A 61-year-woman with long-standing Child A cirrhosis presents with a 24-hour history of abdominal distention and emesis. Last bowel movement was 12 hours ago. Physical examination reveals abdominal distention with hypoactive bowel sounds and a tender mass in the umbilical region. The overlying skin appears to have eschar with minimal fluid weeping. Which of the following is the approach:

a) Emergent repair
b) Elective repair
c) Elastic Velcro abdominal binder.
d) Liver transplantation with repair during transplant.

Patients with symptomatic hernias or those with signs of impending rupture, especially if there is fluid drainage or an eschar, are referred for elective repair. Patients with ruptured or incarcerated hernias should have immediate repair. Patients with asymptomatic hernias are managed conservatively, with surgical correction at the time of liver transplantation. Conservative treatment includes aggressive management of ascites or TIPS if uncontrolled, followed by elective repair. Abdominal binders can also help reduce pain and minimize enlargement of the hernia. **Answer B**.

17) Which of these statements are false regarding hernia repairs:

a) Tension free repairs have lower recurrence rates
b) Ischemic orchitis is a potential complication of inguinal hernia repairs
c) Prosthetic meshes are contraindicated with incarcerated bowel resection
d) The Bassini repair involves the approximation of the transversus abdominis aponeurosis to Cooper's ligament.

Bassini repair involves reconstruction of the posterior wall by suturing the transversalis fascia, the transversus abdominis muscle, the internal oblique muscle, and possibly the iliopubic tract. In **Lichtenstein repair**, mesh is positioned over the inguinal floor. The medial end is secured to the anterior rectus sheath medial to the pubic tubercle. A **Cooper ligament repair** is similar to Bassini, except that the Cooper's ligament instead of the inguinal ligament is used for the medial portion of the repair. Interrupted sutures beginning at the pubic tubercle and continuing laterally along the Cooper's ligament narrow the femoral ring. A transition stitch includes the transversalis fascia, the pectineus fascia, and the iliopubic tract, closing the femoral ring. It also provides a smooth transition to the iliopubic tract over the femoral vessel so that the repair can be continued laterally, as in Bassini. A relaxing incision should always be used given the considerable tension. Ischemic orchitis is caused by over skeletonizing the cord structures leading to venous thrombosis. **Answer D.**

18) Regarding epigastric hernias, all of the following is true, **except**:

a) More common in males
b) Transfascial sutures are necessary
c) Mesh should be used for defects > 3cm
d) Onlay mesh is indicated is diastasis is present

Epigastric hernias are frequently acquired and in obese patients with attenuated tissues. Umbilical hernias are usually considered to be congenital, but many occur later in life and could be considered to result from aging and increases in abdominal pressure. Either an open or laparoscopic repair is possible and mesh reinforcement is nearly always recommended. The method of repair is similar to that of the incisional hernia. Because of the protrusion of abdominal contents due to fascial weakness, patients with diastasis should have their mesh placed intraperitoneally. **Answer D.**

19) Spigelian hernias occur in the following anatomic region:

a) Between the semilunar line and the medial borders of the external oblique, internal oblique, and transversus abdominis muscles
b) Between the semilunar line and the lateral borders of the external oblique, internal oblique, and transversus abdominis muscles
c) Lateral border of the rectus sheath, from the pubic spine to the tip of the ninth costal cartilage
d) Between the umbilicus and the anterior inferior iliac spines

Spigelian hernias usually present with a painless lump in this anatomic area. May also cause incarceration and bowel obstruction. It occurs at the lateral border of rectus muscle through linea semi lunaris because of the posterior sheath absence. Primary repair, mesh placement, open, or laparoscopic are all reasonable options. **Answer A**.

20) Which of the following is false regarding lumbar hernias:

a) Superior triangle (Grynfeltt) is bordered superiorly by the 12th rib
b) Inferior triangle (Petit) is bordered inferiorly by the iliac crest
c) Risk of incarceration is approximately 1-5%
d) Surgical repair should be performed early

Petit's hernia is inferior lumbar triangle hernia with borders of external oblique, latissimus dorsi, and iliac crest. **Grynfelt hernia** is superior lumbar triangle hernia with borders of internal oblique, latissimus dorsi and 12th rib. Lumbar hernias are slow growing with an incarceration risk between 20-30%. They may be repaired by an anterior or posterior approach and small defects can be repaired primarily. **Answer C**.

21) A 78-year-woman with history of complicated sigmoid diverticulitis underwent sigmoidectomy with Hartmans procedure. After 8 months patient develops swelling aroung the colostomy site. Pt now presents to the ER with peristomal pain. Last bowel movement was 12 hours ago. Physical examination reveals abdominal distention with hypoactive bowel sounds and a tender mass in the peristomal area..The overlying skin appears to have erythema and the mass is irreducible. . Which of the following is the false about the patient condition:

a) Patient characteristics that have been associated with an increased risk of PSH formation include obesity, weight gain after ostomy construction
b) Emergency construction of a stoma, chronic or recurrent increases in abdominal pressure have higher association.
c) Mesh repair with stoma translocation is procedure of choice.
d) Primary repair of defect is procedure of choice.

A **parastomal hernia** is a type of incisional hernia that occurs at the site of the stoma or immediately adjacent to it. Placement of ostomy through the rectus muscle is associated with reduced incidence. Prosthetic mesh for construction of a permanent colostomy reduces the risk of hernia formation. Patients with signs and symptoms of ischemic bowel should undergo an urgent or emergent surgical repair.Posthetic mesh use is indicated for patients with symptomatic hernia with recurrent partial small bowel obstruction. The mesh can be inserted laparoscopically or via a laparotomy. Various techniques for parastomal hernia repair have been described, such as Sugar-baker and the key hole technique. **Answer D.**

22) A 78-year-woman with history of complicated right inguinal hernia with 2 hour dissection of chronic direct inguinal hernia. Postoperatively patient complains of severe scrotal pain. Ultrasound of the testis should adequate arterial flow in the testicular artery. Which of the following is the cause of patient's scrotal pain:

a) Subacute orchitis
b) Damage to testis from manipulation
c) Thrombosis of spermatic veins
d) Transaction of vas deference
e) Testicular torsion

Testicular pain after inguinal hernia repair most common results from extensive dissection of the cord to isolate the hernia sac. This may result in damage to the veins of pampiniform plexus in spermatic cord resulting in thrombosis and venous insufficiency As a result it is recommended that surgeon should take gentle care to dissect the sac avoiding trauma to spermatic cod. The sac may be transected at external ring and attempts to excise the sac completely from the scrotum should be avoided.
Answer C.

19. UROLOGY AND GYNECOLOGY

UROLOGY

1) Which of the following stones are the most common after terminal ileum resection/ Ileal conduit:

   a) Struvite
   b) Calcium oxalate
   c) Cysteine
   d) Uric acid

   Besides being the most common kidney stone, incidence increases after terminal ileum resection because of increased colonic absortion of oxalate. Uric acid stones are more common after ileostomy. A hyperchloremic metabolic acidosis occurs in up to 80 percent of patients with ileal conduit. B12 levels are monitored annually beginning three to five years following diversion and that patients are evaluated for symptoms consistent with B12 deficiency. Replacement therapy should be initiated as needed.
   Answer B.

2) 32 year old male presented to your clinic complaining of a painless testicular mass for the past 2 weeks. AFP was elevated and USG did not transluminate. Correct management is:

   a) Fine needle aspiration
   b) Core biopsy
   c) Transinguinal orchiectomy
   d) Trans-scrotal orchiectomy

In any man with a solid, firm mass within the testis, cancer must be ruled out. Prompt diagnosis and treatment provides the best opportunity for cure. Differential diagnosis includes testicular torsion, epididymitis, or epididymoorchitis. Less common problems include hydrocele, varicocele, hernia, hematoma, spermatocele, or syphilitic gumma. USG can distinguish intrinsic from extrinsic lesions, as small as 1 to 2 mm in diameter. A cystic or fluid-filled mass is unlikely to represent malignancy. Radical inguinal orchiectomy is used both to provide the histologic diagnosis and local tumor control. Lesser surgical procedures (biopsy) are generally contraindicated. The initial evaluation should provide information regarding lymphatic spread, the presence or absence of metastases, and the levels of serum beta-hCG and AFP. **Answer C.**

3) Which of the following are the most common cancers in men and women, respectively:

a) Prostate and Breast
b) Prostate and Lungs
c) Lungs and Breast
d) Lungs for both

Most common cancer leading to death is from the lungs. Prostate is second. **Answer A.**

4) Regarding Prostate cancer treatment, which of the following does not constitute an anti-androgen therapy:

a) Etoposide
b) Flutamide
c) Leuprolide
d) Bilateral orchiectomy

The initial evaluation should include clinical staging based upon serum PSA, biopsy of the tumor including assessment of the Gleason score, and DRE. Imaging studies (CT of the abdomen and pelvis, radionuclide bone scan, endorectal MRI) are used selectively to assess for extraprostatic extension, regional adenopathy, or distant metastases. The standard approaches for men with organ-confined T1/T2 cancer are radical prostatectomy (RP), external beam radiation therapy (EBRT), brachytherapy, and active surveillance. Etoposide is a chemotherapy agent used for testicular CA. Options for anti-androgen therapy includes bilateral orchiectomy, anti-androgens (Flutamide) and GnRH analogues (Leuprolide). **Answer A.**

Prostate Ca	Treatment
Localized, low-risk prostate cancer T1	Radical Prostatectomy (RP), External Beam Radio Therapy(EBRT), brachytherapy, and active surveillance
Intermediate-risk disease T1/T2	EBRT, brachytherapy, or RP
High-risk disease T1/T2	Androgen deprivation therapy (ADT) plus EBRT or RP plus adjuvant EBRT
Clinical stage T3 disease	EBRT plus androgen deprivation therapy (ADT) or RP with adjuvant RT
Metastatic prostate cancer	Androgen deprivation therapy (ADT) as the initial systemic treatment

5) 15-yea- old male presented to the ER complaining of acute onset left testicle pain for the past 8hs. USG showed no blood flow to the left testis. Correct management is:

a) Detorsion, antibiotics and scrotal support
b) Bilateral orchiopexy
c) Left orchiectomy
d) Left orchiectomy and right orchiopexy

Testicular torsion results from inadequate fixation of the testis to the tunica vaginalis. If fixation of the lower pole of the testis to the tunica vaginalis is insufficiently broad-based or absent, the testis may torse (twist) on the spermatic cord, potentially producing ischemia from reduced arterial inflow and venous outflow obstruction. Testicular torsion may occur after an inciting event or spontaneously.
It is generally felt that the testis suffers irreversible damage after 12 hours of ischemia due to testicular torsion.
Detorsion and fixation of both the involved testis and the contralateral uninvolved testis should be done. **Answer D.**

6) Where is the urinary collecting system in relation to the renal vessels:

a) Anterior to the renal artery
b) Posterior to the renal artery
c) Anterior to the renal vein
d) Anterior to both the renal artery and vein

The urinary collecting system is the most posterior structure. (Anterior to posterior: Vein, Artery, Pelvis)
Answer B.

7) Which of these statements is false in regards to the renal artery:

a) The right renal artery passes anterior to the IVC
b) The renal artery branches directly off of the aorta
c) The right renal artery is longer than the left renal artery
d) The renal artery branches into four or five segmental vessels.

The right renal artery passes posterior to the IVC.
Answer A.

8) What is the definition of a grade II kidney laceration:

a) Subcapsular hematoma
b) Laceration < 1 cm
c) Laceration > 1 cm
d) Laceration extending into collecting system

A grade II laceration is less than 1 cm and does not extend into the collecting system. When undergoing laparotomy for trauma, the best policy is to explore all **penetrating wounds to** the kidneys. Parenchymal renal injuries are treated with hemostatic and reconstructive techniques: topical methods (electrocautery; argon beam coagulation; application of thrombin-soaked gelatin foam sponge, fibrin glue, or BioGlue) and pledgeted sutures. The collecting system should be closed separately, and the renal capsule should be preserved to close over the repair of the collecting system. Over 90% of all **blunt renal injuries** are treated nonoperatively. Hematuria typically resolves within a few days with bed rest, although rarely bleeding is so persistent that bladder irrigation is warranted. Persistent gross hematuria may require embolization, whereas urinomas can be drained percutaneously. Operative intervention after blunt trauma is limited to renovascular injuries and destructive parenchymal injuries that result in hypotension. **Answer B.**

9) Renal cell carcinomas have been observed to produce all of the following hormones, **except**:

a) PTHrP
b) Erythropoietin
c) Insulin
d) Anti-diuretic hormone

Patients with renal cell carcinoma (RCC) can present with a range of symptoms due to the tumor itself (eg, mass, pain), invasion of the urinary tract (eg, hematuria), paraneoplastic syndromes, or the presence of metastases. Ectopic production of various hormones (eg, erythropoietin, parathyroid hormone-related protein, gonadotropins, human chorionic somatomammotropin, an ACTH-like substance, renin, glucagon, insulin) is common in pt with RCC. **Answer D.**

10) 28 year old Male was brought to the ER after a MVA. Patient was hemodinamically stable despite Hematuria and workup identified a stable pelvic fracture with extraperitoneal bladder injury. Management is:

a) Transurethral Couday catheter placement
b) Percutaneous cystostomy before external fixation of the pelvis
c) Open cystostomy after pelvic fixation
d) Antibiotics and delayed repair in 2 weeks

Bladder injuries are subdivided into those with intra or extraperitoneal extravasation. Ruptures of the intraperitoneal bladder are operatively closed with a running, single-layer, 3-0 absorbable monofilament suture. Laparoscopic repair is becoming common in patients not requiring laparotomy for other injuries. Extraperitoneal ruptures are treated nonoperatively with bladder decompression for 2 weeks. Urethral injuries are managed by bridging the defect with a Foley catheter, with or without direct suture repair. Strictures are not uncommon but can be managed electively. Placement of urinary catheters in trauma patients with Hematuria is contra indicated. Cystostomy should be performed during laparotomy for other reasons or percutaneous if no intervention planned. Complications include stricture and impotence. **Answer B**.

11) 35 year old male s/p ileal resection with short bowel syndrome presents with flank pain and hematuria. KUB reveals radiopaque renal stones, these are most likely from:

   a) Ca phosphate stones
   b) Uric acid stones
   c) Cysteine stones
   d) Ca oxalate stones

Uric acid stones are seen in **gout** and **cysteine stones** are seen in **homocysteinuria**. **Answer D.**

GYNECOLOGY

1) 21 year old female presented to the ER complaining of acute onset RLQ pain for the past 4 hours. Patient became hypotensive and was taken to the operating room. Intra operatively, an unruptured ectopic pregnancy was found. Correct management is:

a) Salpingotomy and unilateral oophorectomy
b) Salpingotomy only
c) Salpingectomy and unilateral oophorectomy
d) Salpingectomy only

Abdominal pain, amenorrhea, and vaginal bleeding are the classic symptoms of ectopic pregnancy. **Ectopic pregnancy** should be suspected in any women of reproductive age with these symptoms, especially those who have risk factors for an extrauterine pregnancy. In women who are hemodynamically stable and appear to have a reasonable probability of future normal tubal function in the affected tube, salpingostomy rather than salpingectomy is recommended. Salpingectomy is indicated in the following situations: uncontrolled bleeding, recurrent ectopic pregnancy in the same tube, severely damaged tube, large tubal pregnancy (ie, greater than 5 cm), and women who have completed childbearing. **Answer B.**

2) 20 year old pregnant in 2nd trimester presented to the ER complaining of RUQ pain and fever for the past 24 hours. USG showed a 1cm appendix with mild periappendiceal fat stranding but no abscess. Correct management is:

a) IV antibiotics and interval appendectomy after delivery
b) IV antibiotic and open appendectomy
c) IV antibiotic and laparoscopic appendectomy
d) IV antibiotic only

The most common general surgery emergency in **pregnancy** is **acute appendicitis**. As the uterus enlarges, the appendix is pushed more cephalad, making the location of pain typically in the RUQ or right flank. U/S may be helpful and is preferred in early pregnancy to avoid the possible teratogenic effects of ionizing radiation. Late in pregnancy, CT can be helpful. Non-perforated appendicitis carries a fetal mortality rate of <5% and perforated appendicitis is associated with a fetal mortality rate 20%. Perforated appendicitis occurs most frequently in the 3rd trimester, when diagnosis can be challenging, again underscoring the importance of early recognition. **Answer C.**

3) During a laparoscopic Nissen fundoplication in a 32 year old female, a 5 cm left ovarian solid tumor was identified. Correct management includes all of the following, except:

a) Tumor biopsy
b) Random omentum biopsies
c) Fluid cytology
d) Total abdominal hysterectomy with bilateral salphingoophrectomy

TAH-BSO should not be performed at initial procedure, particularly in child bearing age. Also the patient has not consented for the procedure which places medicolegal issues forefront. The best thing to do intraoperative is to take biopsy of the mass and proceed with the indicated procedure ie Nissen Fundoplication. **Answer D.**

4) 54 year old female was found to have ovarian cancer involving both ovaries but no lymphnode involvement and distant metastasis. Which of the following corresponds to this patient stage:

a) Stage I
b) Stage II
c) Stage III
d) Stage IV

Stage II is tumor confined to the pelvis, stage III has lymphnode involvement or spread to the abdominal cavity and stage IV has distant metastasis. All stages should have TAH-BSO, omentectomy, lymphnode dissection (pelvic and para-aortic) and biopsies (diaphragm and paracolic gutters) The Gynecologic Oncology Group defines optimal cytoreduction as leaving residual disease less than 1 cm in maximum tumor diameter. All visible tumors should be resected because the volume of residual disease inversely correlates with survival.. If the initial surgical attempt was not optimal, then chemotherapy and secondary surgical cytoreduction may be beneficial, but survival is not as high as with optimal cytoreduction at primary surgery.
Answer A.

5) Which of the following is **not** a risk factor for endometrial cancer:

a) Obesity
b) Multiparity
c) Tamoxifen
d) Early menarche

Following are the risk factor for endometrial cancer: Increasing age, unopposed estrogen therapy, late menopause > 55 yr, nulliparity, obesity, DM, Hereditary non polyposis colorectal cancer, tamoxifen therapy, Family history of endometrial, ovarian, breast, or colon cancer.
Answer B.

6) Oral contraceptive pills are associated with an increase in what type of cancer:

a) Endometrial
b) Cervical
c) Ovarian
d) None of the above

Oral contraceptive pills have been shown to decrease the incidence of endometrial and ovarian carcinomas.
Answer D.

7) The most common trauma seen in pregnant women is:

a) Fall
b) Physical abuse
c) Motor vehicle collision
d) None of the above

In the US, trauma is the leading nonobstetric cause of maternal death. The principal causes of trauma in pregnancy include MVA, falls, homicides, domestic violence, and penetrating wounds. Blunt trauma to the abdomen increases the risk of placental abruption. Once a woman is admitted for trauma, she is at a higher risk for preterm delivery, placental insufficiency, and low birth weight for the remainder of the pregnancy. If discharged undelivered, close outpatient monitoring is warranted with serial growth examinations and antenatal testing depending on the gestational age. Biweekly testing is favored beyond 36 week to improve maternal and fetal conditions. **Answer C.**

8) In the post menopausal women , which of the following is the most common gynecologic cancer:

a) Endometrial
b) Cervical
c) Vulvar
d) Ovarian

The most common endometrial CA is Type I, associated with estrogen stimulation of the endometrium. Type II includes anaplastic, papillary, clear cell, and squamous carcinomas. Treatment usually involves TAH/BSO with lymphadenectomy for type I cancers and for type II, mastectomy is usually added. **Answer A**.

9) 79 year old female was diagnosed with stage I vulvar cancer. Appropriate treatment is:

a) Wide local excision with 1 cm margin
b) Radical local excision with 2 cm margin
c) Radical vulvectomy
d) Radical vulvectomy with ipsilateral lymphadenectomy

Primary surgical treatment for women with all stages of vulvar cancer is the most conservative technique that results in a ≥1 cm tumor-free margin.. Advanced tumors are treated with radical vulvectomy and bilateral lymphadenectomy. Postoperative Radiotherapy to the vulva is recommended for advanced stage, surgically resected patients with high-risk of local recurrence. **Answer B**.

10) Regarding Cervical cancers, which of the following is false:

a) Most commonly associated with HPV types 16 and 18
b) Most cervical cancers are adenocarcinomas
c) Microinvasive cancer can be treated with cone biopsy
d) Stage IIA can be treated with laparoscopic radical hysterectomy and pelvic lymphadenectomy.

Human papillomavirus (HPV) is found to be associated in 99% of cervical cancer. Subtypes HPV **16 and 18** are found in over 70 percent of all cervical cancers. Risk factors for cervical cancer are mostly associated with an increased risk of acquiring or having a compromised immune response to HPV infection; these include: early onset of sexual activity, multiple sexual partners, a high-risk sexual partner, history of sexually transmitted infections, history of vulvar or vaginal squamous intraepithelial neoplasia, and immunosuppression. Oral contraceptive use appears to be associated with an increased risk of cervical cancer. Cigarette smoking appears to be associated with an increased risk of squamous cell cancer, but not adenocarcinoma. The most common histologic types of cervical cancer are squamous cell (70 %) and adenocarcinoma 25 %. **Answer B.**

11) What is the most common cause of intra abdominal bleeding in young females :

   a) Ectopic pregnancy
   b) Liver adenoma
   c) Splenic aneurysm
   d) Ovarian hemorrhagic cyst rupture

   In order of most to least common: 1-Ectopic pregnancy 2- Liver adenoma 3 -Splenic aneurysm. Splenic aneurysms are more susceptible to rupture during pregnancy. **Answer A.**

20. PEDIATRIC SURGERY

1) Which of the following is not part of the foregut:

   a) Lungs
   b) Liver
   c) Bile duct
   d) Duodenum distal to ampulla

   Foregut is composed (besides options a,b and c) by the esophagus, stomach and duodenum proximal to the ampulla. Midgut includes the duodenum distal to the ampulla, the small bowel and large bowel to the distal third of the transverse colon. Hindgut includes distal transverse colon to the anal canal. **Answer D.**

2) 11 year old male, presented to the ED with recurrent vomiting for the past 24hs. Patient weighs 35 kg, correct fluid resuscitation rate is:

   a) 55 ml/h
   b) 65 ml/h
   c) 75 ml/h
   d) 85 ml/h

   Maintenance fluid requirements are calculated by the 4-2-1 rule (4 ml/kg/hr for the first 10 kg body weight, 2 ml/kg/hr for the next 10 kg, and 1 ml/kg/hr for every additional kg). For the first 10 Kg, rate is 4 ml/Kg/hr; for the second 10 Kg, rate is 2 ml/Kg/hr and after that, add 1 ml/Kg/hr. **Answer C.**

3) Which of the following urine output is adequate when resuscitating infants:

a) 0.5 to 1 ml/Kg/hr
b) 1 to 2 ml/Kg/hr
c) 2 to 3 ml/Kg/hr
d) 3-4 ml/Kg/hr

For toddlers and school age, 1ml/Kg/hr is adequate. A newborn should have a urine output of at least 1 to 2 mL/kg/day. **Answer C.**

4) Which of the following is the most common cause of duodenal obstruction in the pediatric population:

a) Annular Pancreas
b) Malrotation
c) Duodenal Atresia
d) Meconium

Duodenal atresia is most commonly seen in newborns and malrotation is seen after this period. **Answer B.**

5) Newborn presented with subacute onset shortness of breath and hypotension for the past 24hs. CXR showed hyperinflation and mediastinal shift. Correct management is:

a) Needle decompression
b) Thoracostomy tube placement
c) Lobectomy
d) Endotracheal tube and Surfactant

Congenital lobar emphysema usually manifests during the first few months of life as a progressive hyperexpansion of one or more lobes of the lung. Air entering during inspiration is trapped in the lobe. On expiration, the lobe cannot deflate and progressively overexpands, causing atelectasis of the adjacent lobes. This hyperexpansion eventually shifts the mediastinum to the opposite side and compromises the other lung. Treatment is resection of the affected lobe using either an open or thoracoscopic approach. Unless symptomatic, resection can usually be performed after the infant is several months old. Ongoing lung development in pediatric patients results in the generation of new alveoli in the remaining lung tissue, unlike in adults. **Answer C.**

6) Regarding pulmonary sequestration, which of the following is correct:

a) Intra-lobar sequestration drains through systemic veins
b) Extra-lobar sequestration drains most commonly through azygous vein
c) Arterial supply most commonly is from bronchial arteries
d) It is not associated with malignancy

Pulmonary sequestration consists of lung tissue not connected to the airway with systemic supply (from thoracic aorta) and intra-lobar drainage through pulmonary veins. In intralobar sequestration the lesion is located within a normal lobe and lacks its own visceral pleura, often presenting with recurrent infections. Venous return is through the pulmonary vein. In extralobar sequestration the mass is located outside the normal lung and has its own visceral pleura. Infectious complications are rare and venous drainage is through systemic veins. Most sequestrations occur in the lower lobes. Elective resection for ILS is recommended because of it's association with recurrent infections. **Answer B.**

7) Which of the following embryologic defect is responsible for umbilical hernia defect formation:

a) Failure of linea semilunares to fuse
b) Failure of linea alba closure
c) Rectus abdominis weakness
d) Failure of transversalis fascia closure

Failure of the umbilical ring to close results in a central defect in the linea alba. The resulting defect is covered by normal umbilical skin and subcutaneous tissue, but the fascial defect allows protrusion of abdominal contents. Hernias less than a centimeter in size at the time of birth usually will close spontaneously by 4 years of life. When the defect is small and spontaneous closure is likely, most surgeons will delay surgical correction until 4 or 5 years of age. If closure does not occur by this time, it is reasonable to repair the hernia. If a younger child has an extremely large hernia, or if the family or child is bothered by the cosmetic appearance, then repair is indicated. **Answer B.**

8) 8 year old male with undescended left testicle should be managed with:

a) Orchiopexy through scrotum incision
b) Orchiopexy through inguinal incision
c) Division of spermatic vessels
d) Unilateral orchiectomy

In **Undescended testis,** the testicle may reside in the retroperineum, and in the internal or external inguinal ring. When the testicle is not within the scrotum, it is subjected to a higher temperature, which results in decreased spermatogenesis. Consequently it is now recommended that an undescended testicle be surgically repositioned by 2 years of age. The administration of HCG occasionally may be effective in bilateral undescended testes, which suggests that these patients are more likely to have a hormone insufficiency than children with unilateral undescended testicle. If there is no testicular descent after a month of endocrine therapy, operative correction should be performed. The operation is typically performed through a combined groin and scrotal incision. The cord vessels are fully mobilized, and the testicle is placed in a dartos pouch within the scrotum.
Answer B.

9) Which of the following is the most common presentation of Wilm's tumor:

a) Hypertension
b) Hematuria
c) Asymptomatic mass
d) Hemi Hypertrophy

Wilms' tumor is the most common primary malignant tumor of the kidney in children which presents as asymptomatic mass. The goal of surgery is complete removal of the tumor. It is crucial to avoid tumor rupture or injury to contiguous organs. A sampling of regional lymph nodes should be included, and all suspicious nodes should be excised or biopsied. Typically a transverse abdominal incision is made, and a transperitoneal approach is used. Provided only unilateral disease is present, a radical nephroureterectomy is then performed with control of the renal pedicle as an initial step. **Answer C.**

10) 2 year old male with known history of Meckel's diverticulum. Most common clinical presentation is:

a) Obstruction
b) Perforation
c) Bleeding
d) Pain

Meckel's diverticulum is a remnant of a portion of the vitelline duct. It is located on the antimesenteric border of the ileum, usually within 2 ft of the ileocecal valve. It may be found incidentally at surgery or may present with inflammation masquerading as appendicitis. Perforation may occur if the outpouching becomes impacted with food. Ectopic gastric mucosa may produce ileal ulcerations that bleed, causing melena. Diagnosis can be made by technetium pertechnetate scans when the patient presents with bleeding. Treatment is surgical. If the base is **narrow** and there is **no mass** present in the lumen of the diverticulum, a wedge resection with transverse closure of the ileum can be performed. A linear stapler is especially useful in this circumstance. When a **mass of ectopic tissue** is palpable, when the **base is wide**, or when there is inflammation, a resection of the involved bowel followed by end-to-end ileoileostomy is preferable. **Answer C.**

11) After birth you examine an infant and notice a 4cm multiloculated, fluctuant mass in the neck. Most likely diagnosis is:

a) Thymoma
b) Branchial cyst
c) Cystic hygroma
d) Sarcoma

Cystic hygroma occurs as a result of sequestration of developing lymphatic vessels. Most common sites are in the posterior triangle of the neck, axilla, groin, and mediastinum. The cysts are lined by endothelium and filled with lymph. These poorly supported vessels may bleed and produce rapid enlargement and discoloration. Infection may occur within the cysts, usually caused by *Strep* or *Staphylococcus*. In the neck this may result in airway compromise. Management of most hygromas includes the combination of surgical excision and image-guided sclerotherapy. Initial treatment typically involves surgery to remove all gross disease without damaging vital structures. Total removal may not be possible because of the extent of the hygroma and its intimate relationship with adjacent nerves, muscles, and blood vessels. **Answer C**.

12) Complications of branchial cleft remnants include all of the following, **except**:

a) Fistula formation
b) Cyst infection
c) External sinuses
d) Cancer

Branchial cleft remnants do not have malignant potential. A fistula is seen most commonly with the 2nd branchial cleft, which normally disappears, and extends from the anterior border of the SCM superiorly, passes inward through the bifurcation of the carotid artery, and enters the posterolateral pharynx just below the tonsillar fossa. In contrast, a third branchial cleft fistula passes posterior to the carotid bifurcation. Remnants may contain small pieces of cartilage and cysts, but internal fistulas are rare. Branchial cleft anomalies occur in association with biliary atresia and congenital cardiac anomalies, an association that is referred to as *Goldenhar's complex*. **Answer D**.

13) The Sistrunk procedure for the removal of a thyroglossal duct cyst includes excision of all except:

a) Lymph nodes
b) Hyoid bone
c) Cyst
d) Tissue below base of tongue

The thyroid gland originates from the base of the tongue in the region of the future foramen cecum at 3 weeks of embryonic life. The "descent" is intimately connected with the development of the hyoid bone. Residual thyroid tissue left behind during the migration may persist and subsequently present in the midline of the neck as a thyroglossal duct cyst. If the duct retains its connection with the pharynx, infection may occur, and the resulting abscess will require incision, drainage, and antibiotics. After resolution of the inflammation, resection of the cyst in continuity with the central portion of the hyoid bone and the tract connecting to the pharynx, in addition to ligation at the foramen cecum (Sistrunk procedure), is curative in >90% of patients. Factors predictive of recurrence include more than two infections before surgery, age <2 years, and inadequate initial operation. **Answer A.**

14) The most common congenital tracheoesophageal fistula is:

a) Proximal tracheoesophageal fistula
b) Esophageal atresia with distal tracheoesophageal fistula
c) Esophageal atresia
d) None of the above

TEF is a common congenital anomaly of the respiratory tract. The diagnosis of EA can be made by attempting to pass a NGT. This finding can be confirmed with an anterior-posterior CXR that demonstrates the catheter curled in the upper esophageal pouch. Type C consists of a proximal esophageal pouch and a distal TEF, which is the most common. Treatment consists of surgical ligation of the fistula and primary anastomosis of the esophageal segments. Primary repair may not be possible if the distance between esophageal segments is large. In that case, staged procedures have been performed that include elongation of the esophagus, gastric transposition, and interposition of the colon. **Answer B.**

15) Which of the following is false regarding hypertrophic pyloric stenosis:

a) More common in Caucasians
b) More common in males
c) Projectile emesis
d) Bilious emesis

Once believed to occur in first-born males between 3 and 6 weeks of age, infants with HPS present with nonbilious vomiting that becomes increasingly projectile over time. Eventually, the infant develops almost complete GOO and is no longer able to tolerate even clear liquids. Despite the recurrent emesis, the child normally has an increased appetite, which leads to a cycle of feeding and vomiting, resulting in severe dehydration. Pyloric stenosis is never a surgical emergency, although the dehydration and electrolyte abnormalities may present as a medical emergency. Fluid resuscitation with correction of electrolyte abnormalities and metabolic alkalosis is essential before induction for operation. After resuscitation, a **Fredet-Ramstedt pyloromyotomy** is performed. The procedure may be performed using an open or laparoscopic approach. **Answer D**.

16) How does the midgut rotate during development:

a) 270 degrees in counterclockwise direction
b) 270 degrees in clockwise direction
c) 230 degrees in counterclockwise direction
d) 230 degrees in clockwise direction

Midgut malrotation - During the 6th week of fetal development, the midgut grows too rapidly to be accommodated in the abdominal cavity, prolapsing into the umbilical cord. Between the 10th and 12th weeks, the midgut returns to the abdominal cavity, undergoing a 270-degree counterclockwise rotation around the SMA. Bilious vomiting is usually the first sign of volvulus, and all infants must be evaluated rapidly to ensure they do not have malrotation with volvulus. If the condition is left untreated, vascular compromise initially causes bloody stools but eventually results in circulatory collapse. Early surgical intervention is mandatory and consists of untwisting counterclockwise. Ladd's procedure basically broaden the mesenteric pedicle to prevent volvulus recurrence. It consists of dividing the bands between the cecum and the abdominal wall and between the duodenum and terminal ileum. This maneuver brings the duodenum into the RLQ and the cecum into the LLQ. Appendectomy is performed to avoid diagnostic errors in later life.
Answer A.

17) Meconium Plug is associated with all of these conditions except:

a) Hirschsprung's disease
b) Crohn's disease
c) Cystic fibrosis
d) Maternal diabetes

The definitive diagnosis of **Hirschsprung's disease** is made by rectal biopsy. A barium enema examination should be performed in children in whom the diagnosis of **Hirschsprung's disease** is suspected. This test may demonstrate the location of the transition zone between the dilated ganglionic colon and the distal constricted aganglionic rectal segment. The treatment for HD is surgical resection of the aganglionic segment of bowel. The normal ganglionic bowel is brought down and anastomosed to the anus, and sphincter function is generally preserved (pull through procedure) Hirschsprung's disease, maternal diabetes, and cystic fibrosis are associated with meconium plugs and may result in intestinal obstruction. **Answer B**.

18) What is the most common cause for intestinal obstruction in a neonate:

a) Hirschsprung's disease
b) Inguinal hernia
c) Intussusception
d) Meconium plug

Intussusception is the most common cause of intestinal obstruction in the neonate, usually in the ileocecal junction. This leads to the development of venous and lymphatic congestion with resulting intestinal edema, leading to ischemia, perforation, and peritonitis. Patients with a typical presentation (sudden onset of intermittent severe abdominal pain with or without rectal bleeding) and stable, may proceed to nonoperative reduction using hydrostatic or pneumatic enema. Surgical treatment is indicated with evidence of perforation, in whom nonoperative reduction is unsuccessful, and/ or for resection of a pathological lead point **Answer C.**

19) Regarding congenital diaphragmatic hernias , which of the following is false:

a) Foramen of Bochdalek is defined as a pleuroperitoneal hiatus
b) Commonly associated with intestinal mal rotation
c) Defect should be repaired immediately
d) Has high mortality

CDH can cause pulmonary hypoplasia, pulmonary HTN, and cardiac dysfunction. Herniation occurs during a critical period of lung development when bronchial and pulmonary artery branching occurs. With worsening lung compression, there is a corresponding decrease in the bronchial branching resulting in a reduction of bronchi and lung tissue. Pulmonary hypoplasia is most severe on the ipsilateral side but may also occur on the contralateral if the mediastinum shifts. Stabilization should be attempted first since early repair has shown to worsen pulmonary function. Persistent pulmonary HTN is the most serious postoperative complication following surgical repair of CDH. **Answer C.**

20) 30 week preterm male child is found to have respiratory distress immediately after being born. On examination, the abdomen is scaphoid. CXR obtained shows following.

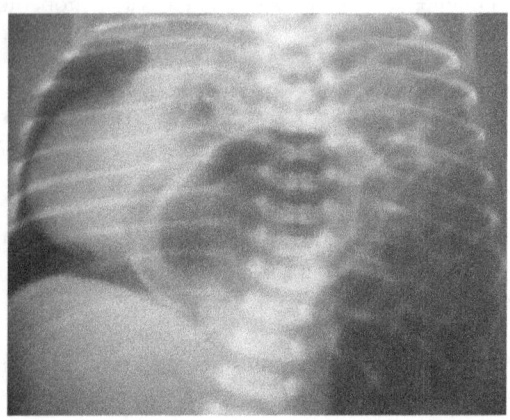

Regarding the most likely diagnosis, which of the following is correct:

a) Preoperative care is directed towards stabilizing the infant's oxygenation, blood pressure, and acid-base status
b) Delayed Surgical correction of hernia is indicated.
c) Immediate NGT placement to decompress the stomach is indicated.
d) Immediate administration of surfactant is indicated to improve pulmonary function.

CDH is a developmental defect in the diaphragm that allows abdominal viscera to herniate into the chest, interfering with lung development. **The morbidity and mortality** of CDH is related to the severity of lung hypoplasia and pulmonary HTN. Infants with CDH most often develop respiratory distress in the first few hours or days of life. The spectrum of presentation can vary from acute, severe respiratory distress at birth, to minimal to no symptoms, which is observed in a much smaller group of patients. Physical examination will reveal a barrel-shaped chest, a scaphoid appearing abdomen because of loss of the abdominal contents into the chest, and the absence of breath sounds on the ipsilateral side. Immediate endotracheal intubation and NGT is indicated to prevent further dilation of abdominal contents. Timing of surgical repair remains unclear and is dependent on the severity of the respiratory distress. Bochdalek hernia occurs posterior to the left while morgagni hernia occurs anteriorly (retrostenal). The diagnosis of diaphragmatic eventration is made when there is abnormal displacement of part or all of an intact diaphragm into the chest cavity. **Answer D.**

21) A 10-year-old boy complains of severe pain in the scrotum. Examination of the scrotum shows a tender right testis, which lies higher than the left. The most appropriate management is:

a) Scrotal ultrasound
b) Right groin exploration
c) Bilateral orchiopexy
d) Warm compression.

Detorsion and fixation (open book technique) of both the **involved** testis and the contralateral **uninvolved** testis should be done since inadequate fixation is usually a bilateral defect. Longer periods of ischemia may cause infarction of the testis requiring orchiectomy. **Answer C.**

22) A 7 days old, healthy girl has abdominal pain, mild jaundice. Ultrasonography shows dilation of intrahepatic bile duct with triangular cord sign. Which of the following is the next step in management:

a) HIDA scan
b) Liver biopsy
c) Ursodeoxycholic acid
d) Intraoperative cholangiogram

A liver biopsy in indicated all infants with suspected biliary atresia. Histologic changes consistent with biliary atresia warrant immediate Kasai procedure. Patency of the extrahepatic biliary tree can be further assessed by hepatobiliary scintigraphy. Failure of tracer excretion suggests Biliary Atresia. If the above measures fail to support diagnosis of biliary atresia, intraoperative cholangiogram is done. If contrast doesnot reach the intestine, Diagnosis of Biliary atresia is confirmed and Hepatoportoenterosotomy (Kasai) procedure is done. **Answer B.**

23) In a healthy 1-year-old child who is 12 kg, comes in with dehydration. the maintenance fluid requirement is:

a) 52 cc/hr
b) 44 cc/hr
c) 62cc/hr
d) 50cc/hr

Maintenance fluid requirements are calculated by the 4-2-1 rule (4 ml/kg/hr for the first 10 kg body weight, 2 ml/kg/hr for the next 10 kg, and 1 ml/kg/hr for every additional kg). For 12 kg child, 40 cc/hr + 4cc/hr = 44 cc/hr. **Answer B**.

24) 4 months old male is found to have a left neck mass. Rotation of the head toward the right side makes it prominent. Which of the following is most likely the diagnosis:

a) Thymoma
b) Branchial cyst
c) Cystic hygroma
d) Torticollis

The presence of a lateral neck mass in infancy in association with rotation of the head toward the opposite side of the mass indicates the presence of congenital **torticollis**. This lesion results from fibrosis of the sternocleidomastoid muscle. The mass may be palpated in the affected muscle in approximately two thirds of cases. Histologically, the lesion is characterized by the deposition of collagen and fibroblasts around atrophied muscle cells. In the overwhelming majority of cases, physical therapy based on passive stretching of the affected muscle is of benefit. Rarely, surgical transection of the sternocleidomastoid muscle may be indicated. **Answer D.**

21. NEUROSURGERY AND ORTHOPEDICS

1) Which of the following is false regarding cerebral saccular aneurysms:

   a) Associated with polycystic kidney disease
   b) Occur at branch points in the arteries
   c) Defect in intima layer
   d) The likelihood of multiple aneurysm is 20%

   Intracranial saccular aneurysms are thin-walled protrusions composed of a very thin tunica media, and a severely fragmented internal elastic lamina. All symptomatic aneurysms should be considered for treatment with relative urgency. Small aneurysms (<7 mm) in patients without previous SAH, observation is generally advocated. Special consideration for treatment should be given to young patients. Asymptomatic aneurysms ≥7 to 10 mm warrant strong consideration for treatment, taking into account patient age, medical and neurologic conditions, and relative risks for treatment. **Answer C.**

2) The normal range for intracranial pressure is:

   a) 0 to 5 mmHg
   b) 5 to 15 mm Hg
   c) 15 to 30 mmHg
   d) 30 to 40 mmHg

ICP is normally ≤15 mmHg in adults, and pathologic intracranial hypertension (ICH) is present at pressures ≥20 mmHg. Cerebral perfusion pressure (CPP) is a clinical surrogate for the adequacy of cerebral perfusion. CPP is defined as mean arterial pressure (MAP) minus IntraCranial Pressure (ICP).

CPP = MAP – ICP

Conditions associated with elevated ICP, including mass lesions and hydrocephalus, can be associated with a reduction in CPP. CPP should be kept between 60 and 75 mmHg in patients with elevated ICP, in an attempt to avoid hypoperfusion and ischemic injury. **Answer B**.

3) 30 year old male was seen in your office 2 weeks after a MVA and crush injury to his right upper extremity. Patient complaints of loss of sensation in the affected extremity. Which of the following is the correct nerve regeneration rate:

a) 0.1 mm/day
b) 1 mm/day
c) 0.1 cm/day
d) 1 cm/day

Nerve regeneration may occur if the axon is injured but the myelin sheath is preserved. **Neurapraxia** is the least severe form of nerve injury, with complete recovery. In this case, the actual structure of the nerve remains intact, but there is an interruption in conduction of the impulse down the nerve fiber. Most commonly, this involves compression of the nerve or disruption to the blood supply. There is a temporary loss of function. **Axonotmesis** is disruption of the **neuronal axon** with maintenance of the **myelin sheath**. It may cause **paralysis** of the motor,**sensory**, and **autonomic**. **Neurotmesis** is the most severe lesion, not only the axon, but the encapsulating connective tissue loses their continuity. The last degree of neurotmesis is transsectionThere is a complete loss of motor, sensory and **autonomic** function. Nerve regeneration occurs at rate **1mm/ day. Answer B.**

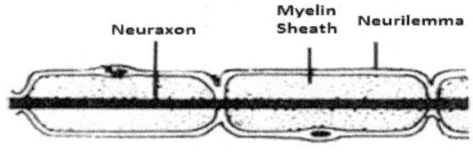

Myelinated Nerve fiber

4) Which of the following spinal cord lesions is characterized by loss of ipsilateral motor function and contra-lateral loss of pain and temperature sensation below the level of injury:

a) Brown-Sequard syndrome
b) Complete cord transection
c) Cauda Equina syndrome
d) Spinal shock

Brown-Séquard syndrome is a loss of sensation and motor function caused by the lateral hemisection of the spinal cord.
Symptoms: Loss of pain and temperature sensation on contralateral side of body.
Central cord syndrome is characterized by loss of pain and temperature sensation   at the site of the spinal cord lesion which is caused by the disruption of   spinothalamic fibers in the anterior commissure.
Anterior spinal artery syndrome usually includes tracts in the anterior two-thirds of the spinal cord, which causes bilateral loss of pain and temperature sensation. Tactile, position, and vibratory sensation are normal. Urinary incontinence is usually present.   Complete cord transection is characterized by areflexia, anesthesia and flaccid paralysis; **Cauda equina** presents with weakness in lower extremities and loss of bladder or bowel function. **Spinal shock** includes hypotension with warm extremities. **Answer A.**

5)   48 year old female presents to your office complaining of pain and decreased movement of the right thumb. Which of the following nerve is affected in this syndrome:

a) Radial
b) Ulnar
c) Median
d) Musculocutaneous

Carpal tunnel syndrome occurs when the median nerve is compressed at the wrist.

Nerve	Sensory	Motor	Injury
Median	Palmar side of the thumb, the index and middle finger, half the ring finger	Lumbricals 1 & 2, thenar eminence	Ape hand deformity
Ulnar	Fifth digit and the medial half of the fourth digit, and the corresponding part of the palm	Interossei (Dorsal-Abductor **DAB**, Palmer-Adductor **PAD**)	Claw hand
Radial	Back of the hand, including the web of skin between the thumb and index finger.	Extensors of Hand and digits	Wrist drop/ Saturday night palsy

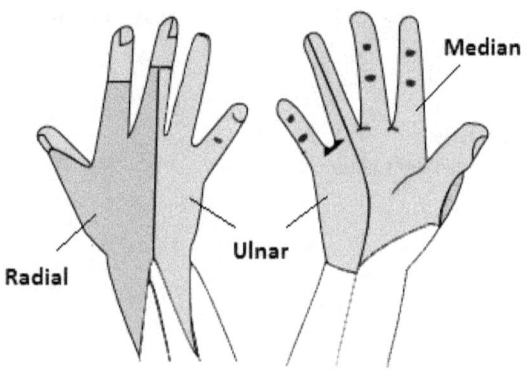

Answer C.

6) Which of the following fractures is not associated with avascular necrosis:

a) Femoral neck
b) Clavicle
c) Talus
d) Scaphoid

Clavicle and 5th metatarsal fractures are associated with non union. Delay in treatment of Clavicle and Femoral neck fractures leads to avascular necrosis. **Answer A.**

7) 27 year old male was brought in to the ER after a MVA. Patient complaints of right shoulder pain, which was anteriorly dislocated. Structure most likely to be injured is:

a) Axillary artery
b) Axillary nerve
c) Radial artery
d) Radial nerve

Axillary nerve may be injured during anterior shoulder dislocation which leads to decresed sensation of lateral shoulder and decrease deltoid strength (arm abduction). **Radial nerve injury** is associated with mid-shaft humeral fracture affecting the extensors of wrist and finger causing wrist drop. Supracondylar fracture of the humerus causes brachial artery injury causing ischemic necrosis of flexor muscles of forearm causing permanent flexor contracture of hand and wrist, known as **Volkman's ischemic contracture. Answer A.**

8) 28 year old male s/p being assaulted and hit with a baseball bat, presented to the ED with left supracondylar fracture. Orthopedics performs closed reduction and 24hs post op, patient complaints of pain and hypoesthesia in the forearm. Most likely cause is:

a) Brachial artery injury followed by reperfusion
b) Radial artery injury followed by reperfusion
c) Ulnar artery injury followed by reperfusion
d) Anterior interosseous artery injury followed by reperfusion

Volkmann's contracture occurs after supracondylar fracture associated with anterior interosseous injury and reperfusion after reduction. Patients develop compartment syndrome in the forearm and treatment indicated is volar and dorsal fasciotomies. **Answer A.**

9) 49 year old female presented to your office with a history of recently being diagnosed with Carpal tunnel syndrome. Initial management includes all of the following, **except**:

a) Steroid injections
b) Splinting
c) Non steroid anti inflammatory
d) Carpal ligament release

Initial conservative management of carpal tunnel syndrome includes Splinting, glucocorticoids injected into the carpal tunnel, and oral glucocorticoids. For patients with severe carpal tunnel syndrome that is refractory to conservative measures, surgical decompression is recommended.
Answer D.

10) 30 year old male presented to the ER 24hs after hitting his left hand against the window. Patient was complaining of pain with passive motion and had tendon sheath tenderness during palpation. Correct treatment is:

a) Admission and IV antibiotics
b) PO antibiotics and follow up as outpatient
c) Wound debridement and steroids
d) Antibiotics , longitudinal incision and drainage

Suppurative tenosynovitis may occur after minor traumas and involves proximal spread into the tendon sheath. It usually results in closed space infection of flexor tendon sheath which can spread to deep spaces of palm. Physical examination is significant for erythema and tenderness along the course of the sheath. Patients hold the wrist in flexion as active or passive extension provokes intense pain. Early surgical intervention with open or closed irrigation of the sheath remains the "gold standard", as treatment with antibiotics alone is rarely successful. **Answer D.**

11) 61 year old male is complaining of right hip pain after hitting the dashboard during a MVA. Most common associated injury is:

a) Femoral artery
b) Femoral nerve
c) Sciatic nerve
d) Obturator nerve

Posterior hip dislocations usually caused by a motor vehicle accident with the passenger's knee hitting the dashboard and forcing the femoral head out of the acetabulum posteriorly. The limb is shortened, and the hip flexed, the foot is in internal rotation Posterior dislocation of the hip is associated with sciatic nerve lesion, and anterior dislocations are associated with femoral artery or nerve injuries. With an anterior dislocation the lower limb is lengthened, the hip abducted and the foot is in external rotation. As the femur head is either anterior in the groin or in the obturator fossa it can obstruct the femoral vein causing thrombosis and possible pulmonary embolism.
Answer C.

12) 42 year old male was hit during a soccer game and presented to the ED with posterior knee dislocation. Management includes all of the following, **except**:

a) Angiogram
b) Duplex USG
c) ABI
d) ORIF

The most common mechanism of injury for a posterior knee dislocation is a direct force on the tibia when the knee is flexed, forcing the tibia posteriorly on the femur. This mechanism primarily occurs when the tibia strikes the dashboard or when a runner falls on a flexed knee Posterior dislocation should be treated with closed reduction immediately due to higher incidence of popliteal artery injury. Vascular studies are indicated to rule out popliteal artery injury. The presence of an ABI of < 0.9 is both highly sensitive and specific for the diagnosis of arterial injury associated with knee dislocation, suggesting that routine angiography does not seem to be necessary in patients presenting with knee dislocation. ABI < 0.9 after knee dislocation warrants angiography/CTA as they are associated with higher incidence of arterial injury.
Answer D.

13) 53 year old male, s/p MVA and popliteal artery injury was revascularized 6 hs later. Next day patient developed compartment syndrome in the affected extremity and foot eversion after fasciotomies. Most likely injured nerve is:

a) Common peroneal nerve
b) Superficial peroneal nerve
c) Deep peroneal nerve
d) Tibial Nerve

Compartment syndrome is a limb-threatening condition frequently caused by long bone fracture, vascular injuries, burns, crush injuries, intravenous infiltration. The earliest and most important symptom is pain out of proportion and severe pain at rest or passive stretching. Medial and lateral incisions are done for fasciotomy to decompress all four compartments of leg. Most commonly injury structures during fasciotomy are saphenous vein and superficial peroneal nerve. **Answer B.**

14) 74 year old female was complaining of acute onset respiratory distress after her femur fracture repair. Patient developed confusion and Sudan red stain was positive. Correct treatment is:

a) Endotracheal tube placement and IV heparin drip
b) Thrombolytic therapy
c) IVC filter placement
d) Oxygen therapy and ICU admission

Fat embolism is usually associated with long bone and pelvic fractures. It presents usually 24-72 hours after intial injury as dyspnea, hypoxemia, and tachypnea. Neurologic abnormalities with altered level of consciousness are also seen. Characteristic petechial rash is last component of the triad (hypoxemia, neurologic abnormality, petechial rash). Treatment is supportive but may require intubation in severe cases. **Answer D.**

15) Regarding lower extremity anatomy, which of the following structures is not located in the deep posterior compartment of the leg:

a) Sural Nerve
b) Tibial Nerve
c) Posterior tibial artery
d) Peroneal artery

The Sural nerve is located in the superficial posterior compartment. The anterior compartment contains the anterior tibial artery and the deep peroneal nerve and the lateral compartment contains the superficial peroneal nerve. **Answer A.**

16) Which of the following symptom is the first present in compartment syndrome:

a) Pain
b) Edema
c) Paresthesia
d) Decreased temperature

ACS can occur in any anatomic compartment bound by fascial membranes. The lower leg is a common site and is comprised of 4 compartments. Signs and symptons include : Pain with passive motion (early finding), tense compartment, pallor, diminished sensation, weakness, paralysis (late finding). Normal pressure usually falls between 0 and 8 mmHg. Capillary blood flow becomes compromised at 20 mmHg, pain develops between 20 and 30 mmHg, and ischemia occurs above 30 mmHg. Immediate management includes relieving all external pressure, limb should NOT be elevated, analgesics and O2 should be given. Fasciotomy is the definitive treatment and delays may increase morbidity. Compartments are the anterior, lateral, deep posterior, and superficial posterior, with the anterior being the most commonly affected. Loss of pulse is an ominous and late finding. **Answer A.**

17) 71 year old male presented to your office after noticed a mass in his right thigh. Biopsy was performed and confirmed osteosarcoma. Most important prognostic factor is:

a) Lymphnode involvement
b) Mitotic rate
c) Age
d) Tumor grade

Osteosarcoma is the most common primary malignant tumor of bone Sarcomas spread hematogenously and tumor grade is the most important prognostic factor . Surgery and systemic chemotherapy are the mainstays of treatment for patients with osteosarcomas and other primary bone tumors such as malignant fibrous histiocytoma and fibrosarcoma. Although there is no specific survival benefit to preoperative as compared to postoperative chemotherapy in osteosarcoma patients, the neoadjuvant approach may permit a greater number of patients to undergo limb-sparing procedures. However, chemotherapy is no substitute for sound surgical judgment when assessing the need for amputation versus limb-sparing surgery. The optimal chemotherapy regimen has not been established.
Answer D.

18) 38 year old male presented to the ED with pain in the right finger for the past 24hs. You examined and diagnose paronychia. Correct treatment is:

a) Incision and drainage
b) Bilateral incision
c) Warm compress and antibiotic
d) Nail removal

Paronychia is suggested by a swollen and tender nail folds. A purulent collection is often present and it must be distinguished from **felon**, an infection of the digital pulp characterized by severe pain, swelling, and erythema. Treatment of **felon** requires emergent incision and drainage to prevent osteomyelitis, nail deformities, and ischemic necrosis. Therapy of acute paronychia without abscess includes local care. When abscess is present, incision and drainage should also be performed. **Answer C.**

19) 59 year old male presented to the ED 6hs after MVA with open fracture of the mid-femur. Correct treatment is:

   a) Closed reduction and internal fixation
   b) ORIF
   c) Open reduction and external fixation
   d) Antibiotics, debridement and transmedullary metal rod placement

   Midshaft femur fractures are most commonly caused by high energy trauma. Surgery is indicated because of the high rate of union, low rate of complications, and the advantage of early fracture stabilization. For trauma patients with severe concomitant injuries, early definitive repair is associated with higher morbidity. Open fractures should be repaired with external fixators and left open because of the high infection rate. Definitive repair, usually with IM nailing, is delayed for approximately five days, until the patient is stabilized. **Answer C.**

20) 20 year male presented to the ED after a MVA complaining of RLE pain. Physical exam showed an adducted and medially rotated right lower extremity. Most likely injury is:

   a) Anterior hip dislocation
   b) Posterior hip dislocation
   c) Femur fracture at the neck
   d) Femur fracture at the proximal aspect

Anterior dislocation usually presents with lateral rotation. With an anterior dislocation the lower limb is lengthened, the hip abducted and the foot is in external rotation. As the femur head is either anterior in the groin or in the obturator fossa it can obstruct the femoral vein causing thrombosis and possible pulmonary embolism.

Posterior hip dislocations are the most common. The usual cause is a motor vehicle accident with the passenger's knee hitting the dashboard and forcing the femoral head out of the acetabulum posteriorly. The limb is shortened, and the hip flexed, the foot is in internal rotation. Sciatic nerve damage is common – which affects the dorsiflexion of the foot. **Answer B.**

21) Regarding disk herniation, which nerve is most likely to be involved at the L4-L5 level:

a) Sciatic nerve
b) Femoral nerve
c) Common peroneal nerve
d) Tibial nerve

Most cases of disk herniation involve the L4-L5 and L5-S1 level. Common peroneal nerve is usually involved with L4-L5 disk herniation and presents as ipsilateral weakness and foot eversion.

C5	Elbow Flexion
C6	Wrist extension
C7	Elbow extension
C8	Finger flexion
L2	Hip Flexors
L3	Knee extensors
L4	Ankle dorsiflexion
S1	Ankle plantarflexion

Answer C.

22) Which of the following is false regarding shoulder dislocations:

a) 95% are anterior dislocations
b) Posterior dislocation are associated with seizures
c) Axillary nerve palsy may be present
d) Reduction can usually be achieved with internal rotation

A blow to the anterior portion of the shoulder, axial loading of an adducted and internally rotated arm, or violent muscle contractions following a seizure or electrocution represent the most common causes of **posterior shoulder dislocation**. **Anterior dislocations** are usually caused by a direct blow to or fall on an outstretched arm. The patient typically appears holding their arm externally rotated and slightly abducted.It can result in damage to the axillary artery and axillary nerve (C5, C6). Damage to the axillary nerve results in a weakened or paralysed deltoid muscle. Reduction can usually be achieved with gentle external rotation of the arm. **Answer D.**

23) What is a type B pelvic fracture:

a) Non-displaced fracture
b) Vertically unstable fracture
c) Rotationally unstable fracture
d) None of the above

In **type A injuries**, the sacroiliac complex is intact. The pelvic ring has a stable fracture that can be managed nonoperatively. **Type B injuries** are caused by either external or internal rotational forces resulting in partial disruption of the posterior sacroiliac complex. These are often unstable. **Type C injuries** are characterized by complete disruption of the posterior sacroiliac complex and are both rotationally and vertically unstable. These injuries are the result of great force, usually from a motor vehicle crash, fall from a height, or severe compression. **Answer C.**

24) Which of the following is false regarding renal trauma:

a) Grade V renal trauma includes complete parenchymal shattering
b) Penetrating trauma is more severe than blunt trauma
c) Penetrating trauma is more common than blunt trauma
d) Grade V renal trauma includes vascular avulsion

Blunt trauma accounts for 90% of renal trauma. **Answer C.**

25) 25 years old male was admitted to ER after falling from the roof in upright position. Commonly associated fractures include, **except**:

a) Cervical spine fracture
b) Calcaneous fracture
c) Wrist/forearm fracture
d) Lumbar fracture

Cervical spine fracture is usually associated with axial loading and distraction and extension injuries. Lumbar spine fractures are usually compression (wedge) type fractures. **Answer A.**

22. STATISTICS

1) Regarding Type II error , which of the following is true:

   a) Incorrectly rejects the null hypothesis
   b) Assumes that no difference exists between groups
   c) Assumes there was no difference when it actually exists
   d) Occurs commonly due to large sample size

   Option A describes a Type I error, option B describes the Null hypothesis and Type II can be better identified with larger sample size. **Answer C.**

2) Which of the following parameter best measure central tendency when there are no outliers in a set of values:

   a) Mean
   b) Mode
   c) Median
   d) Confidence interval

   Mode is the most frequent value and median is the middle value of a set of data. **Answer A**.

3) The number of patients in Brazil with Dengue fever in the summer of 2014 is an example of:

   a) Prevalence
   b) Incidence
   c) Odds ratio
   d) Relative risk

   Incidence is the number of new cases in a specific time frame and prevalence is the number of patients with the disease. **Answer A.**

4) Which of the following studies effectively avoids observational bias:

a) Meta-analysis
b) Case-control study
c) Randomized controlled trial
d) Double-Blind controlled trial

Although RCT's are also prospective studies, it avoids treatment bias. **Answer D**.

5) Which of the following tests is characterized by qualitative variables analysis:

a) Paired t-test
b) Chi-squared test
c) ANOVAs
d) Student's t-test

The other options are quantitative tests. Non parametric statistics and Kaplan Meier estimator are also examples of qualitative tests. **Answer B**.

6) Which of the following options describes sensitivity:

a) Patients with the disease and positive test
b) Patients without the disease and positive test
c) Patients with the disease and negative test
d) Patients without the disease and negative test

Sensitivity is the proportion of patients with the disease who test positive, measuring the ability to detect the disease. **Answer A**.

7) Which of the following options describes specificity:

a) True negatives / False positive + True negative
b) True negative / False negative + True negative
c) False positive / False negative + True negative
d) True positive / False positive + True positive

Specificity is the proportion of patients without the disease who test negative, measuring the ability to confirm there is no disease. **Answer A**.

8) Which of the following statistical measures determines the likelihood of not having a disease with a negative test result:

a) Specificity
b) Sensitivity
c) Positive predictive value
d) Negative predictive value

Positive predictive value is the patient population with the disease who has positive results. **Answer D.**

9) Which of the following statistical values does not depend on the disease prevalence:

a) Sensitivity and Specificity
b) Sensitivity and Positive predictive value
c) Specificity and Negative predictive value
d) Positive and Negative predictive values

Predictive values depend on prevalence. **Answer A.**

10) Regarding preventive medicine, screening colonoscopy is a type of:

a) Primary prevention
b) Secondary prevention
c) Tertiary prevention
d) Quaternary prevention

Primary prevention is used to avoid the disease, such as immunizations; Secondary prevention are those tests used to detect disease early , such as mammograms and pap smear ; Tertiary prevention is used to lower the morbidity of an established disease, such as DM and HTN control. **Answer B.**

11) As of 2014 the state of Texas has a 30-35% of the population with Obesity. This statement would represent:

a) Incidence
b) Prevalence
c) Relative risk
d) Rate of disease
e) Odds ratio

Prevalence represents the number of people with a disease in a population at a given time. Incidence = new cases only. **Answer B.**

12) A study is undertaken to analyze the effects of the "*Bacalhau Syrup*"on reducing stress among surgical residents. All of the statistical data has been found to be significant for the effect, but when given to the residents was not found helpful. This phenomenon would represent:

a) Variance
b) Type II error
c) Type I error
d) Confidence interval
e) Median variation

Type I error occurs when the null hypothesis is rejected when is actually true, in other words, assuming that there is a difference or effect when actually no difference exists. The chance that the findings are not true is represented by the *p value*. Type II error is the opposite, in which we assume there is no benefits when there actually is. Increasing power may help reduce type II errors. **Answer C.**

13) In a residency program consisting of 20 residents, 7 of them answered 75% of all the questions correct, while 5 answered 63%, 6 of them answered 45% and 2 of the residents answered 85% of all questions correct. The mode and mean would be respectively:

a) 75%, 64
b) 45%, 75
c) 63%, 62
d) 85%, 71
e) 65%, 68

The mode is the most frequent value. Since the majority of residents scored 75 this would represent the mode. The mean is the average and when added all scores and divided by the number of residents will yield the mean. **Answer A.**

14) The residency program directors of a busy university hospital with more than 200 residents are conducting a prospective study from May through August of the present year to assess the effects of resident's lab coat cleanliness and the development of surgical site infections. The project was presented in April during one of the combined interdisciplinary conference among residents and faculty. This study design could lead to potential bias due to:

a) Reporting bias
b) Lead-time bias
c) Sampling bias
d) Hawthorne effect
e) Detection bias

The Hawthorne effect is form of response whereby subjects improve or modify an aspect of their behavior being measured simply in response to the fact that they know they are being studied. The residents will likely show up with clean lab coats during the months of May thru August. **Answer D.**

15) A new screening modality for the detection of colon cancer is being implemented. The subjects of the study were also evaluated by colonoscopy and CT. The test was found to have a sensitivity of 99% with a specificity of 45%. A negative result will likely represent:

a) Is likely a false negative
b) More than likely is a true negative
c) True positive rate is low
d) Accuracy is 95%
e) A positive result means the patient have colon CA for sure.

A very sensitive test has a great ability to detect individuals with the disease, but may also label patients without the disease as positive when they are not. In contrast, a negative result is very likely to be a true negative and therefore very unlikely to have the disease. **Answer B.**

*The ABSITE Exam

* "The ABSITE consists of approximately 225 multiple-choice questions. The exam is administered solely online and it is presented in one five-hour block".

*"The ABS has decided to merge the junior and senior level exams into one exam starting 2014".

*"The ABS provides the ABSITE to all ACGME-accredited general surgery residency programs. It is also made available to osteopathic, international programs, and to integrated vascular surgery residency programs"

*From the American Board of Surgery website. For more information, go to: http://www.absurgery.org.

NOTES